Living the Therapeutic Touch

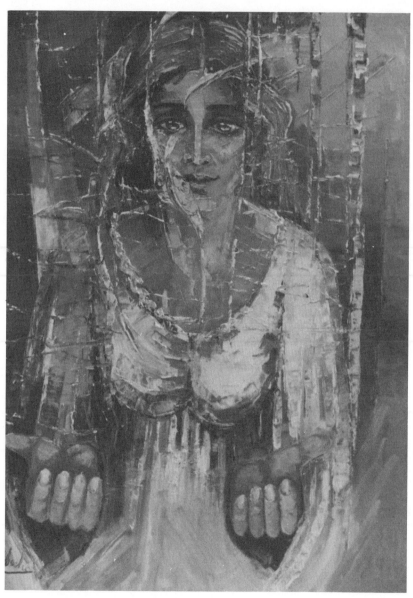

The Compassionate Mother of the World. An artistic interpretation by Nabeela George.

Living the Therapeutic Touch

HEALING AS A LIFESTYLE

Dolores Krieger, Ph.D., R.N.

Dodd, Mead & Company
New York

No part of this book may be reproduced in any form
without permission in writing from the publisher.
Published by Dodd, Mead & Company, Inc.
71 Fifth Avenue, New York, N.Y. 10003
Manufactured in the United States of America

First Edition

1 2 3 4 5 6 7 8 9 10

Library of Congress Cataloging-in-Publication Data

Krieger, Dolores.
  Living the therapeutic touch: healing as a lifestyle / Dolores
Krieger.
     p. cm.
  Bibliography: p.
  Includes index.
  ISBN 0-396-09025-7
  1. Mental healing. 2. Vital Force—Therapeutic use. I. Title.
RZ401.K74 1987
615.8′51—dc 19

                                             87-20898
                                              CIP

Dedicated to Emily B. Sellon,
who encouraged me to seek out
my own interpretation of life and living
but, as should all opinion,
"hold it in your hand, but lightly."

CONTENTS

List of Appendices   ix
List of Tables   xi
Acknowledgments   xiii
Introduction   xv
Chapter 1: The Persistent Reality   1
Chapter 2: Transitional Stages   17
Chapter 3: A Yoga of Healing   35
Chapter 4: The Healing Act as an Experience
            in Creativity   65
Chapter 5: Therapeutic Use of the Paranormal   75
Chapter 6: Therapeutic Touch as
            an Evolutionary Emergent   103
Chapter 7: Healing as a Lifestyle   113
            Appendices   125
            Notes   189
            Index   197

LIST OF APPENDICES

Appendix A: "Listening" to Oneself: A Tool for Self-Awareness **125**

Appendix B: Visualization of the Dance of Energy Forms **127**

Appendix C: Exploration of Personal Field Dynamics **129**

Appendix D: Exploration of Others' Field Dynamics **131**

Appendix E: Human Field Holomovement **134**

Appendix F: Vivid Visualization: Review of the Literature and Theoretical Rationale **136**

Appendix G: Vivid Visualization: Statistical Analysis **142**

Appendix H: Vivid Visualization: Nurse-Meditator's Form **147**

Appendix I: Vivid Visualization: Nurse-Observer's Form **151**

Appendix J: Therapeutic Touch During Childbirth Preparation by the Lamaze Method and its Relation to Marital Satisfaction and State Anxiety of the Married Couple **157**

Appendix K: Therapeutic Touch During Childbirth Preparation: Definition of Terms **159**

Appendix L: Therapeutic Touch During Childbirth Preparation: Delimitations of the Study, Hypotheses, and Research Question **161**

Appendix M: Therapeutic Touch During Childbirth Preparation: Significance of the Study **163**

Appendix N: Therapeutic Touch During Childbirth Preparation: Review of the Literature **164**

Appendix O: Therapeutic Touch During Childbirth Preparation: Methodology, Research Findings, and Discussion **167**

Appendix P: Therapeutic Touch During Childbirth Preparation: Explanation Offered to Persons Whose Permission is Requested **175**

Appendix Q: Therapeutic Touch During Childbirth Preparation: Consent Form **176**

Appendix R: Therapeutic Touch During Childbirth Preparation: Subjective Experience of Therapeutic Touch Scale (SETTS) **177**

Appendix S: Therapeutic Touch During Childbirth Preparation: Protocol for Teaching Therapeutic Touch to Husbands **184**

LIST OF TABLES

Table 1: Summary of Hemoglobin Values of Six Subjects Who Were Treated by the Laying-On of Hands and Two Controls Over Very Short Periods of Time **14**

Table 2: Summary of Before and After Hemoglobin Values of Three Subjects Who Acted as Their Own Controls **15**

Table 3: Raw Data of Nurse-Meditators in Experimental Group on Measures of Hits, Misses, and Items Not Perceived on Each of Two Patients **92**

Table 4: Raw Data of Professional Nurses in Control Group on Measures of Hits, Misses, and Items Not Perceived on Each of Two Patients **93**

Table 5: Multiple Fisher's t Test Re: Differences Between the Uncorrelated Means of Data on Perceptions of the Three Experimental Small Groups **143**

Table 6: Analysis of Variance of Data on Hits in the Three Experimental Small Groups and F Ratios **144**

Table 7: Analysis of Variance of Data on Misses in the Three Experimental Small Groups and F Ratios **144**

Table 8: Analysis of Variance of Data on Items Not Perceived in the Three Experimental Small Groups and F Ratios   **145**

Table 9: Fisher's *t* for Testing a Difference Between Uncorrelated Means of Experimental Group as a Whole and the Control Group on Hits, Misses, and Items Not Perceived   **145**

Table 10: Means and Standard Deviations for Hits, Misses, and Items Not Perceived for Experimental Group as a Whole and the Control Group   **145**

Table 11: Pearson's Product Moment Coefficient of Correlation of Patient #1 and Patient #2 in the Experimental Group on the Measures of Hits, Misses, and Items Not Perceived, and *t* Ratio for Testing the Significance of Each Coefficient of Correlation   **146**

Table 12: Analysis of Pretest Scores on the Interpersonal Conflict Scale   **171**

Table 13: Analysis of Pretest Scores on STAI   **171**

Table 14: Analysis of Posttest Scores on the Interpersonal Conflict Scale   **172**

ACKNOWLEDGMENTS

*F*oremost, I would like to express my appreciation to Ms. Dora Kunz, who opened my eyes to the healing way; Ms. Emily Sellon, to whom I have dedicated this book, and then to my many friends, colleagues and students who have provided the constant challenge. I also want to express my appreciation to Lynne Lumsden for her insightful editorial support that lent eloquence to what had been mere words, to Nabeela George, for permission to reproduce her abstract painting, *The Compassionate Mother of the World*, to Leila Mowad for her poem, "Reflections of Therapeutic Touch," and to Betsy Ungvarsky, for her delightful time lapse photograph of myself healing myself.

INTRODUCTION

*T*his book is very much my own interpretation of how the ordering principles that underlie the healing process can become a centering focus in the ever-transforming mandala (a patterned wheel or circle of concepts or symbols) of one's life. This personal perspective has been molded over the past eighteen years through an intensive study of the healing process and through the development and teaching of Therapeutic Touch, which I undertook together with my teacher, Ms. Dora Kunz. Therapeutic Touch is an ancient healing modality cast into the contemporary mode. At this time it has been taught in thirty-eight countries in addition to the United States. As one might expect, much of my experience in healing is in reference to Therapeutic Touch; however, from discussions with many healers in several countries, there is a common core relevant to all healing practices. Specific directions for the practice of Therapeutic Touch are included in the Appendix. However, if you want a deeper discussion and demonstration of the techniques, I would suggest that you read *The Therapeutic Touch: How to Use Your Hands to Help or to Heal*‡, which I wrote a few years ago, or *Clinical Implications of Therapeutic Touch*, which will be published in 1988.

Living the Therapeutic Touch

CHAPTER ONE

The Persistent Reality

*T*here is a strange phenomenon that may occur in the lives of those who study in depth various modes of healing. It very frequently happens that, after the researcher's studies have demonstrated the validity of the healing (as a therapeutic mode distinct from allopathic, traditional, medicine), the researcher often reports a personal need to learn how to heal. The persistence of the reality of man's ability to help presses upon the researcher with an unusual urgency to know for him or herself. This curious occurrence appears to act in reverse to a principle well known in the new physics, Heisenberg's principle of complementarity. Heisenberg's principle states that a scientist's observations in themselves are enough to change the phenomena being studied. The opposite effect happens in reference to healing: When the researcher studies the phenomenon (healing), the phenomenon changes the researcher. This frequently acts to shape a significant transformation in the researcher's lifestyle, as experiences in helping or healing others deepen.

Healing as a lifestyle is not a miracle way; it is hard work. The conviction that healing others is a natural potential, which I firmly believe, does not minimize the fact that this potential can be realized only in a climate that nourishes basic needs of others. To remain healthy in such an environment, the healer must couple that consideration for others with a wholesome recognition of one's own needs. Within this matrix of concern the healer demonstrates a commitment to healing, and his or her lifestyle is declared.

THE BREAKING DOWN OF BARRIERS

Sensitivity to the needs of others as well as the frank recognition of one's own needs have come into vogue only recently. The major thrust in this direction occurred between 1965 and 1975, as many Western populations were exposed to a variety of non-Western cultures. Masses of people traveled to non-Western countries in unprecedented numbers. This people-to-people experience broke through many attitudinal barriers that had been carefully erected in the name of economic, social, political, territorial and national self interests. Along with this personal introduction to other cultures and traditions came recognition of realities that were not based on the accepted norms of the Western world, but that had nevertheless persisted for centuries in other cultures.

Interestingly, during the same ten-year time frame, the mating of high technology with the life sciences, such as biology and neurology, began to give credence to the existence of facets of human consciousness previously unrecognized, and in many cases unsuspected, by Western science. The pioneering procedure here was biofeedback. Biofeedback is a psychotechnologic procedure. A person is telemetered to highly sophisticated electronic devices that read out, or "feed back" data (either through visual information or as changes in the intensity of light or the pitch of audible tones), on the present state or level of that individual's physiological processes. The therapeutic use of this information involves a little-understood maneuver in the individual's internal consciousness, whereby that person can learn to alter the readings on the machine's monitor and thereby gain control of one or more physiological processes. Biofeedback regulation or reinforcement has been extended to the autonomic nervous system (once thought to be impervious to voluntary control), to encephalographic and musculoskeletal responses, and to procedures that significantly influence mood and emotion.[1]

This high-tech therapeutic form has been a major instrument for the validation of alternate and multiple realities of the yogi[2] and the shaman.[3] The translation of these ancient teachings about self into a Western jargon has made the accompanying practices available to those of us born in this materialistic and pragmatic culture. Our culture makes available large measures of physical comfort, intricate psychological rationalizations and complex generalizations about life and the universe. But our standardized perspective on reality does not provide adequate answers to fundamental questions regarding a satisfying human existence: *How can I make my life more meaningful? In what way can my life make the universe more meaningful to others?*

These are the questions I asked myself during this time period. These are the concerns that haunt the person who feels committed to the life-affirmative: to help people who hurt or are in discomfort; to help those who don't know how to focus their own capabilities for self healing; to help those who have to live with limitations to seek out their own courage and to live fully within those confines; to help such persons find avenues of healthful, creative expression in other facets of their being and, when the appropriate time approaches, to help the dying person go through the passages of release to other states of consciousness. Such is the temper of people who want to help others. These concerns fire the drive of those who feel impelled to heal.

During the subsequent ten years, 1975 to 1985, the impetus toward a new understanding of the potentialities of human consciousness, which had been initiated by the psychotechnologies, found unexpected support and supplementation from science. The precursor of this outpouring of new models was the application of systems theory to the analysis of human function and human behavior.[4,5] This strategy brought into focus the importance of context and the recognition of the interrelatedness of all things. The clarification and generalization of the new physics led to the recognition of significant correlations between theoretical implications of the new physics, and the teaching of ancient oriental philosophies.[6,7]

Interdisciplinary study became more acceptable. One of the major successes of such cooperative effort was the acknowledgment of psycho-physio-neuroimmunilogical bases of stress and the consequent appreciation that stress-related disorders are pandemic in our world.[8] To counteract this scourge of our time, across the country swept a rising tide of popular interest in therapeutic modes that could neutralize the deleterious effects of stress. One result of this avid interest was the growth of a loosely organized grassroots movement, called holistic health, which attempted to see the individual within his or her unique context.[9] Holistic health advocates mainly supported activities that facilitated a relaxation response, an integrated set of physiological responses that opposes the fight-or-flight reaction to stress and promotes the body's restorative processes.[10]

A fuller view of human potential came into focus. This perspective indicated the validity of other ways of knowing, and an unparalleled search for this new knowledge and the personal growth it ensured surged spontaneously across socioeconomic and educational lines. Too new and too radical for the formal classroom, this new knowledge was taught in workshops and conferences, seminars and discussion groups, and indeed wherever the interested would gather. The quality of the teachings and the teachers was mixed, but the need to know was clear. Where individuals were able to personally synthesize these new ideas, the resulting shift in awareness frequently provided a ground against which previously murky, unresolved questions could be answered.

In her brilliant psychohistory of the current paradigm shift, *The Aquarian Conspiracy*,[11] Ferguson describes the major stages of this human transformation. This shift provides the conditions for the acceptance of the healer in Western culture at this time in history. The essential stages of Ferguson's model follow the individual from the time of his or her first exposure to the new perspective, through a stage of increasing interest in the introductory information, to new and different ways of using one's consciousness and, finally, to an effort towards the integration of this new knowledge into one's lifestyle. Specifically considered, they are:

1. **Entry point.** The introduction of the person to the new knowledge. Here, there is a realization of another deeper, more provocative and interesting way of perceiving life than what is usual in our rational and prosaic culture. Within this perspective life has a more personal meaning to the individual. For the healer, this stage frequently comes with the recognition that, contrary to traditional beliefs, he has access to an overabundance of human energies and that he can learn to direct and modulate them in the act of being therapeutic to self and to others.[12] This confrontation with other realities can be profoundly unsettling. Ferguson describes the state: "Here the unfettered mind suffers a kind of agoraphobia, a fear of its own awesome spaces."[13] Nevertheless, the individual may persist and go on to the second stage.

2. **Exploration.** A deliberate search for experiences that will help restructure one's life around the perspective of the new knowledge.

The new knowledge interfaces with many systems of thought, both ancient and modern. Therefore, the search demands discrimination, as well as perserverance, as the healer pursues this personal growth experience. He or she may begin to realize that answers are not to be found in any single approach, since they are unique for each of us. If the answer is to be found at all, it will arise in the working through of the question—the quest itself. This now-acknowledged need for introspection may lead one to the third, and final, stage.

3. Integration. When one realizes that within one's self is both the path—the seeking—as well as the source of what is sought, his or her personal search may be refocused. The searcher may then begin to seek out the deeper structures of his or her own being. As the functions of these structures are acknowledged, they provide the background against which the learned facets of the new knowledge unite. In this unique patterning they become one's own.

Working through these perceptions of the new consciousness heightens awareness of one's own frailties as clearly as it demonstrates strengths. Therefore, a seeking out of modalities for self healing is frequently initiated with the search for other philosophical perspectives. Under the best of circumstances, these two avenues of inquiry may lead to a further synthesis. This might work out as follows: A basic assumption of the new knowledge is that the individual is a multifaceted consciousness. Every aspect is, by its very nature, related to every other aspect. Each dimension of consciousness has the potential to affect the person as a whole unified being.

This wholeness is not only greater than the sum of its parts, it is different. It is this nexus of connectivities that lends structure to both the individual and to his or her environment. Therefore, it is in this arena of interaction between these two that the basis for human function is formed. When these relationships are in dynamic balance, the person is in a state of health or well being. Each individual possesses an inborn capacity for self healing, and each human being has access to an innate potential for self-transformation.

If the individual really accepts these assumptions, the logical conclusions regarding health become apparent. We each have personal control over our own state of being, but we must also accept individual responsibility for its condition. Those who are not in optimal health seek out therapeutic modes that will not only help them regain that control, but provide a means to understanding that acknowledged responsibility. It is a curious fact that, under these circumstances, when a conscious attempt is made to fully engage the functions of the inner self in the activities of daily living, quite often a healing of that person will occur.

Whether or not healing has occurred, persons who consciously draw upon the functions of the self during times of crisis may gain unexpected insight into their illness. Such resolution may significantly alter their perspective on life. Healers agree that many of their former patients have experienced such an irresistable urge to share insights or healings that they have learned some therapeutic modality so that they, too, can help or heal others in distress. Here, from an unanticipated source, one witnesses the imprint of the persistent reality of healing as it indelibly marks the lives of those who have shared its experience.

What is involved in the healing act that it can have such profound effects on the lifestyle of both healer and healee? Although there are many different healing styles (perhaps as numerous as the many different ways we as human beings can compassionately relate to one another), in general, the healing act is a conscious, full engagement of one's energies in the interest of helping another person. Both the intention and the motivation of the healer, and the healee's acceptance of the illness and his willingness to change, serve to deepen and temper the healing act in an individual way. Contrary to expectations, both repeated studies and clinical evidence of a variety of healing methods strongly indicate that there is no significant correlation between the degree of a healee's faith in getting well and whether that person will in fact be healed.[14]

THE HEALING ACT

What are the actual dynamics of the healing act? To date there is very little measurable evidence concerning the highly personalized energy interaction that takes place between healer and healee. Either present technology is not "high" enough or, more likely, its lexicon of data relates to a very different universe of discourse than mere numbers suggest. The actual dynamics of the healing act remain largely conjecture. In 1980, after more than a decade of active involvement in research, clinical practice and the teaching of healing, I developed a theory about the healing act based upon these experiences.

My major involvement in healing has been concerned with Therapeutic Touch, which Dora Kunz and I derived from the ancient practice of laying-on of hands, but which is not identical to it. Unlike the laying-on of hands, for instance, Therapeutic Touch does not have a religious context; its techniques were built upon intensive research and modern teaching strategies. Also, in Therapeutic Touch healing is regarded as a natural human potential. It is not reserved for the chosen few. In addition, Therapeutic Touch is not necessarily a "hands-on" modality. In many of its techniques the healer's hands do not come into direct contact with the healee's body.

Therapeutic Touch could be called a human field phenomenon; that is, much of the hypothesized energy transfer occurs outside the periphery of the healee's body, in his/her energy field or personal surroundings. Subsequent experiences with and study of many other types of healing appear to affirm my suppositions.

I state this conceptualization as follows. Human beings are open systems. They appear to be a nexus of all fields of which life partakes. That is, human beings are the energetic matrices of inorganic as well as organic fields, psychodynamic as well as conceptual fields (i.e., electromagnetic is only one interface of the whole complex). Human beings are therefore exquisitely sensitive to wave phenomena (i.e., energy). I perceive the healer to be an individual whose personal health gives him access to an overabundance of *prana* for the well-being of others. (Prana is a Sanskrit term for what we in the West think of as the organization of energy that underlies the life process.) Prana is concerned with the intrinsic rhythmicity of energy, as *kundalini* (to be discussed later. For definition, see p. 44) is fundamentally concerned with consciousness.

Using deductive logic I re-examined my previous studies in the life sciences. It occurred to me that at the physical level, this projection of human energy during the healing act grounds itself in the ill person via electron transfer resonance. The resonance acts in the service of the ill person to reestablish the vital flow in this open system. It restores unimpeded communication between the individual's field complex and the environment. Given this, as all literature on healing agrees, the healees then actually heal themselves.

Further theoretical analysis of this model suggested the possibility that if the healee was able to sustain this threshold (i.e., if the healee's own recuperative powers were adequately activated), full recovery could be achieved. If the integrity of the healee's system was too fragmented to respond once it was on its own, that person's recovery would be less complete. After an initial spurt there could be a relapse, or there might not be any apparent effect.[15]

Although Therapeutic Touch is a way of helping and/or healing that is derived from the prehistoric practice of the laying-on of hands, it also differs from this practice in that it neither has a religious context, nor does it depend on the faith of the client for its effects. Therapeutic Touch has been built upon a growing base of substantive research findings[16-25]. It is known that its effects are replicable. Its teaching has been developed within the context of validated contemporary teaching strategies.

This documented base has enabled Therapeutic Touch to be taught, at this writing, in more than eighty universities and colleges. It is also taught in innumerable hospital in-service programs in the United States, and in more than thirty-eight foreign countries. Nationally and internationally the hospital in-service programs can be viewed via the Hospital Satellite Programs, and the current listings of literature on Therapeutic Touch can be called up through the computer program MEDLINE.

According to Stone Age pictographs found in the Pyrenees, man's ability to heal is exceedingly ancient—at least 15,000 years old. The practice of healing, probably initiated to protect the strength of clan or tribe, has been found in the traditions and customs of all people. Through the centuries the life-giving or healing energies have been called by various names in different parts of the world, and many of these names continue in use. Prana, mentioned above, flows through conductor circuits called *nadis* in Sanskrit. The Egyptian word for these energies at the psychophysical level is *ka*. In Chinese it is the *ch'i* (*Qi* in Pinyon), in Tibetan it is called *ylun*, and the Kahunas of Hawaii call it *mana*.

In spite of differences in language and symbolic structures, there are many major points of agreement about the function of these energies. As you shall see in Chapter 3, many non-Western cultures have conceived a system of intricate mechanisms for processing these life-sustaining energies in human beings. This understanding has been developed in its most subjectively sophisticated form in the East (specifically in India, Tibet, China and Japan). In Sanskrit these complex structures, which are non-physical, are called *chakras*. In our terms, chakras are roughly analogous to electronic transformers. They transform or step down the significant energies in the environment to energy states that make us what we are as human beings.

For most of us, except under unusual conditions, the functioning of these chakras occurs below the level of conscious awareness, much like the activities of the autonomic nervous system on the physical level. As the healer gains more experience in healing, an increasing sense of the farther reaches of consciousness may move some healers to sharpen their sensitivity to these subtle functions with the conscious intent of learning to use them upon demand.

What does this prana feel like to the healer? Since prana is a natural means of energizing all life processes, the "feeling" of pranic flow is not much different than the normal sense of wellbeing known to those in a high state of health. But if one is willing to become aware of the subtleties of that state, one senses that all bodily functions are exquisitely synchronized. The timing of events in one's life, in retrospect, seems uncanny, and, as will be discussed in fuller detail in Chapter 5, there is an increase in psychic abilities. Further, if the deeper emotional and cognitive structures of the self are engaged during the healing act in experiences of interiorization, acts of intuition and creativity become more firmly meshed in one's lifestyle as the more profound level of prana yields its secrets to the inquiring mind.

INTERIORITY

Even in primitive cultures there is ample evidence that healing is closely allied to an inner, more subtle life. Katz, writing on healers among the !Kung of the Kalahari Desert, says: "Healers are more involved (than the general population) in their own inner processes, more open to the unfamiliar both within and outside themselves. Yet, while they are open to their inner processes, they are able to control them."[26] And Elkin describes Australian aboriginal healers as professional persons of special training who "seek knowledge through quietness and receptivity, meditation and recollection."[27] These descriptions of earnest involvement in introspection find agreement among healers of diverse cultures. The *manambal*, the indigenous healers of the Philippines; the *izinyanga*, Bantu curers in South Africa; and the *curandero* of Central America describe their healing experiences as acts of interiority.

Although there is general agreement on this personal knowledge, it is nonetheless a cultural world view and individual life experience that colors the healer's own conception of the dynamics of the healing act. For instance, there is no clear concensus on the source of healing energy. Some healers think the source is of their own making, others claim it arises out of some universal power source, such as God. A different point of view is that the healing energies are invested in and focused by one's ancestors. There is also the universally recurring notion of invisible allies—archetypal figures who emerge from nonphysical realms to communicate with the healer or to invest the healer or medicinal plant or object with healing power.

In addition, the personal nature of this experience in interiorization makes it difficult to translate into everyday language. In talking to an anthropologist about her healing work, WaNa, an aged healer among the !Kung, says, "I don't know whether to tell others about the details of my *NUM* [a unique type of energy flow through which her healing ability comes forth during transcendent states of consciousness] . . . These things I am talking about are very difficult things and a different way of living."[28]

HEALERS IN HISTORY

However they may interpret their own experiences, it is evident that something marks healers as different from other people. Landy remarks that the reason ethnologists have paid so much attention to healers is that they are very often the most striking and knowledgeable personages in the group under study. He says, "Observers were greatly impressed by the complexities of individual healers and the wide variation in implementation of the role of healer."[29]

Because of the unusual character of many healers, several have become legendary. Romano, for instance, tells about the widespread fame of a 19th century Mexican healer even during his own lifetime. After his death he was apotheosized by the Roman Catholic Church and attained the status of a religious folk saint.[30]

History records many famous people who had healing abilities.

Cuniform tablets tell of the healing ability of Thrita, a physician from ancient Persia. Ancient texts attest to the ability of Dhen-Wantari, a physician of India, and of Galen of Greece, physician to Macus Aurelius, who also was a well known healer. In ancient Greece, Hippocrates himself advocated the use of the laying-on of hands, and Pliny reports that a case of snakebite was cured by this method.

Royalty was thought to carry healing power, and the early kings and queens of England and France were renowned for their ability to cure goiter and other throat conditions. The Roman Emperor Hadrian was said to be able to reduce "dropsy" (a condition of abnormal accumulation of fluid in body tissues and cavities that can accompany heart disease, cirrhosis of the liver, and some kidney diseases). The Emperor Vespasian was noted for his ability to therapeutically intervene in neurological disorders, conditions of lameness and blindness.

There are forty-one citations of healing in the New Testament. Pope Alexander III issued an edict in the 12th Century against the healing mission of clergy. But history records a large number of priests who acted upon Jesus' teaching to go out and heal the multitudes. In Ireland St. Patrick healed the blind by touch, and in France St. Bernard is known to have healed a variety of infirmities—blindness, lameness, muteness, and deafness—in the congregations of Cologne.

In the West, the recognition of laypersons who could heal, and who could convince authorities of the validity of their treatments has, until quite recently, had scant notice. When I was in England, the work of Valentine Greatrakes, a 17th century Irish landowner and magistrate, was brought to my attention.[31]

Since he is one of the few in Western history to have been viewed in a positive light, it is useful to review his record. After some years spent in the service of Oliver Cromwell, Greatrakes returned to his home in Ireland and, for unrecorded reasons, he became interested in the laying-on of hands. With practice, Greatrakes found that he could produce a therapeutic effect without actually touching the patient's body. (This fact much surprised me, for I thought that healing without direct body contact was something we had developed in Therapeutic Touch!) This was very important for Greatrakes's time since it obviated the need to remove a patient's clothes for treatment. Among the records of his healings were instances of paralysis, deafness and headaches. It is said that the swellings of tumors and the inflammations of arthritis also disappeared.

There is recorded evidence of Greatrakes's highly successful and widely reported healing tour of London in 1666. Moreover, he published a description of his methods, including detailed case histories. He admitted that his methods were not always successful and, being a man of some wealth, he refused payment for his treatment. These factors and his position in Anglo-Irish society, along with the fact that he publicly stated that the healing force could only come from God, insured that accusations of witchcraft (common at that time) were never directed against him. Nonetheless, physicians refused to pay attention to him and silently ignored his findings. Eventually, Greatrakes quietly returned to his estate, leaving the medical profession—and, more importantly, the people—all the poorer for not having taken this opportunity to learn from someone whose only interest was to help others.

TOWARDS NEW CONCEPTS OF RESEARCH ON HEALING

In Western society there is a long history of refusal to acknowledge healing modalities that do not—perhaps because they cannot—fit into the mechanistic confines of empirical science. Today, for those who have been made aware of the dynamics of scientific revolutions, there is little basis for continuing such a stance. If the highly personalized nature of the healing act escapes the mesh of contrived logic and artificially controlled methodologies of Western science, then we should look to the modeling of that network for possible errors or misfit.[32] The "anomaly" should not be cast aside out of hand. Even sophisticated multivariate statistical analyses do not catch the subtle nuances of human interaction. If we are to truly understand how humans relate, we need new models and new modes of imaging for both our research designs and our repertoire of analytic ploys.

In the late 1960s, in a serious attempt to assist in such a change, I planned to study the effect of laying-on of hands on certain physiological indices, specifically the blood components, hemoglobin and blood plasma. It turned out to be the first controlled, substantive study done on physiological factors during the healing of human beings. There was no recipe for such an undertaking. Therefore, I had to create my own models. Nevertheless, both the validity and the reliability of this research have withstood rigorous critique over the years.

In this study I was looking at the effect that treatment by the laying-on of hands might have on the hemoglobin value. This is concerned with the iron in the blood, and the hematocrit ratio, which computes the proportion of the red blood cells (which contain the iron molecule) to other components in the blood. It is the hemoglobin molecule that carries oxygen to the cells of the body. I chose to look at these phenomena because human beings have an oxidative metabolism. Oxygen transport is central to the basic building up and breaking down of body cells in the life process, which is itself a prime definition of healing.

Using samples adequate in size and composition to permit complex statistical analyses, the research findings supported a hunch I had that treatment by the laying-on of hands would change the healee's blood components. In the Experimental Group there were significant changes in both the hemoglobin values and the hematocrit ratio. However, in the matched Control Group, where laying-on of hands was not done, both the hemoglobin values and the hematocrit ratios remained unchanged. Technically, the level of confidence in that finding was $p < .01$, a value of considerable statistical significance. Although the hemoglobin values and hematocrit ratios consistently tend to increase following the laying-on of hands (and also in later studies with Therapeutic Touch that were built on this pioneer effort), in the many years we have refined the initial study, there has never been any indication from the data that the laboratory findings exceeded normal range. I have never made the claim that these increases in blood levels indicated that healing had occurred. Nevertheless, the fact that these components have stayed within normal limits gives a hint of the ordering principles that underlie the healing process.

Two of the factors that appear to be important to this ordering principle are time and timing. In reference to time, it seems that healing occurs best while the illness is in its early stages, before there has been extensive organic damage. However, time itself seems to be different during the healing process. Change may occur very quickly. As can be seen on Table 1, the blood components themselves demonstrate very rapid change, perhaps reflecting the accelerated change going on as part of the healing process itself.

Table 1 highlights changes that occurred in hemoglobin values over very short periods under research-controlled conditions in six patients (Subjects #1 to #6) in a subsample of the study noted above. Blood samples were drawn before and after they had been treated with the laying-on of hands. The changes that occurred in hemoglobin value, all of which occurred in less than one day, are significant. In contradistinction, there is no change at all in the two Subjects (#7 and #8) who were not treated. The changes in the Experimental Group were stable and maintained those levels for the entirety of the research period. Later research in which Therapeutic Touch, rather than laying-on of hands, was the treatment modality demonstrated the same stability. Note in particular the time-matched pairs, Subjects #3 and #7 and Subjects #2 and #8, on Table 1. Over the matched periods Subject #2 changed 1.5 Gms., while there was no change in #8. The comparable change in Subject #3 was 0.8 Gms. of hemoglobin but, again, there was no change in #7's hemoglobin values.

Timing is as important in healing as it is in the internal synchronization of bodily activity or in the latency of family genetic

---

TABLE 1

Summary of Hemoglobin Values* of Six Subjects Who
Were Treated by the Laying-On of Hands and Two
Controls Over Very Short Periods of Time

Subject	Medical Diagnosis	Period Between Blood Samples	Hemoglobin Values Before	After
#1	GI Disorder	22 hours	13.3	12.5
#2	Nervous exhaustion	18 hours	9.4	10.9
#3	Metastatic cancer	45 minutes	14.1	14.9
#4	Nervous exhaustion	6 hours	12.5	14.1
#5	Endocrine imbalance	22 hours	14.1	14.9
#6	Cataract, left eye	6¼ hours	14.1	15.6
#7	Control	45 minutes	13.3	13.3
#8	Control	18 hours	13.3	13.3

*Grams per 100ml. blood

traits. These are traits that one is born with, but which may not be apparent until specific times in later life when conditions are appropriate. Like these genetic traits, a number of circumstances must come together for healing to occur with ease.

Table 2 can serve to further strengthen the notion of the important relationship between timing and healing. Table 2 illustrates a very small portion of the original sampling, three persons who were originally in the Control (untreated) Group for six days. During this time they were, of course, subjected to all the pertinent conditions as were the Experimental Group. However, there was no change in the laboratory findings of their blood components. These same persons, who were ill, were then treated with the laying-on of hands by a healer. As can be seen by the figures on the extreme right side of Table 2, subsequent significant change occurred in their hemoglobin values. These early studies that I did between 1969 and 1974 have been replicated by others in the United States and abroad with similar findings. Further data can be found in the Proceedings of the 9th Conference of Nursing Research of the American Nurses Association (see Chapter 1, note 16). The rapidity of physiological change under these circumstances suggests that within the context of healing, time itself may dance to a different beat than our usual tick-tock chronology.

TABLE 2
Summary of Before and After Hemoglobin Values of Three Subjects Who Acted as Their Own Controls*

Subject	Medical Diagnosis	Control		Experimental	
		Pretest	Posttest	Pretest	Posttest
A	Bone displacement	9.4	10.1	10.1	15.6
B	Hypoglycemia	12.5	12.5	12.5	14.9
C	Psychological Disorder	14.1	14.1	14.1	14.9

*In essence, the Control posttest hemoglobin values are the same as the Subject's pretest values when the subject is later transferred to the Experimental Group and treated.

THE PERSISTENT REALITY

Research is but one basis for reality. Life itself provides an irrefutable experiential base to our concepts of reality. In the relationship we call the healing act, it is obvious from the powerful changes that frequently occur in the experienced healer's life (and which may also occur in the life of the healee), that deep, core structures of the self may be stimulated to enter into and affect everyday life activities. This transfer of the locus of control of personal behavior to the inner core of being is important to the well-being of a society that values actualization of the potential of the self. The persistent reality of the healing act can activate compelling life-affirmative drives in those who heal. Surely it is worth the attention of our most astute minds, as well as those who are merely compassionate.

Experiencing the persistent reality of the mature and committed healer offers access to the most highly regarded values of our human civilization. These values are very similar to those expressed by subjects involved in Maslow's study of the process of self actualization.[33] Like the self actualizers, healers report critical changes in self image. They also report changes in the way they relate to the world in general and to the people with whom they personally interact. They are responsive to creativity, spontaneity, expressiveness and idiosyncracity in themselves and in others. They sense meaningfulness in life because they have touched the more subtle reaches of its nature during their peak experiences of helping others.

These times of greatest maturity, individuation and fulfillment, of actualizing their greatest human potentialities (events that Maslow has called "their healthiest moments") are regarded by them as highly desirable. They then want to repeat the experience. These moments of high-level consciousness are, of course, the end products of attunement to the compelling urgencies of a persistent reality. What are the significant signposts of this transformative process and how can we make them part of our own experience of "healthiest moments?" We now direct our attention to the transitional stages that occur in the lives of those who strive to heal self and others.

CHAPTER TWO

Transitional Stages

*W*hy do people want to help or to heal others? Sympathy, empathy, or compassion is the motivation for this most humane of human acts. Curiously, however, none of these traits are considered necessary survival skills in the long evolution of humanity. Why, then, do they persist? This question cannot be pursued very far before it gives rise to a gnawing hunch that there are significant gaps in what we know about the human condition.

THE WOUNDED HEALER

Among the human thinking patterns psychologists call archetypes, there is a constellation known collectively as the Wounded Healer. Archetypes have their own inner logic, whereby the materials of our consciousness are structured in a characteristic manner. They convey, through symbol and image, not only the intention, but also the direction, and probably the meaning, of the process in which they are involved. Ira Progoff writes:

> As a proto-image the archetype is present in principle at the very beginning of the process, and that is why it is a fact that dreams very frequently reveal an unconscious foreknowledge of the path of development that will unfold in the future in an individual's personality.[34]

Moreover, he points out that in the Jungian view each archetype is thought to have the capacity for infinite development and differentiation.

17

There are two basic interpretations of the Wounded Healer. One version has an individual who has been ill, wounded or otherwise traumatized. This person experiences his or her own healing by healing others. Every healing of another results in a symbiotic self-healing of one's own wounds. Ultimately, this leads the Wounded Healer to a realization of the profundity of the process of being healed, of being made whole. A sense of at-oneness may occur while he or she is engaged in the healing act. Here, there is conscious recognition that others are also fundamentally at one, whole, even though they may be ill, wounded or weakened. With conscious recognition of this fundamental similarity, the Healer reaches out to heal.

Another version of the Wounded Healer is an individual who has suffered, but who has decided to help others so that they need not undergo the pain and weakness, the discomfort and dependency of similar suffering. This compassionate intent points toward the model for compassion that is known in Buddhism as the Bodhisattva vow. In this tradition, an individual who has completed the fullness of human evolution and attained spiritual enlightenment may leave this world of pain and sorrow for other higher realms of consciousness, achieving a state of perpetual bliss. The bodhisattva, however, renounces this personal salvation, vowing to remain in this world until all other beings have reached a similar state. It is from the depths of this compassionate grace that transformation occurs.

THE NOVICE HEALER

Most impulses toward healing others lie somewhere along the spectrum between these two versions. If they persist steadily over time, the result is frequently a significant restructuring of the self. At the time of this writing, I have taught different modes of healing to more than 16,000 professionals in the health field. Most of my teaching has been of Therapeutic Touch.[35] The journals of these students reveal a significant consistency. At first, the novice healer is paralyzed with self-doubt and has difficulty making a commitment. If they are willing to put aside this fear of possible failure, students realize that the important thing is to try to help others in need. When one learns something new, the effort is frequently accompanied by a certain amount of awkwardness. But if the novice can hold fast to the primary intent, which is to meet the needs of the patient, the ego's desire to succeed will fall into perspective. Moreover, once the novice healer discovers that it is really possible to help, there is a shift in self-image and in self-worth. Consequently, relationships with others are perceived differently. The journal of a student states the case cogently:

"As a nurse administrator, I have not had 'hands on' in a clinical situation for the past three years. As all nurse administrators at our hospital do, I pitch in now and then in the intensive care unit and help out. One can get very rusty very quickly, but there are aspects of care-giving that stay with you always: the overwhelming feeling of wanting to help the ill and the dying. Recently, I was asked to help in the intensive care unit. The unit was very busy, and I knew they had admitted a teenage girl who had been in an automobile accident on the thruway. I went to the unit and suddenly was aware of a perceptible 'pull' toward the girl's room. I asked the head nurse if I could care for this patient. She agreed and I went immediately to the young girl's bedside.

She looked smaller than her fourteen years. She lay twisted, and her body twitched with pain each time she tried to move. She tried desperately to smile at me, but her eyes told me the horror and pain she was now feeling. My first thought was: I really don't know what I can do for this child except meet her immediate clinical needs. Since the first day of class, every day I have carried with me the thought of healing and/or helping someone in severe discomfort or pain. But now as I looked at her the question *What can I really do?* sent a wave of nausea through me. . . .

Sitting in the darkened room, I wondered, *Who do I really want to help?* Did I want to help this child, to try to relieve some pain and increase her comfort? Did I want her to sleep through the day? Or was this for me, so that I could have some peace of mind? Did I want to use her to prove to myself that Therapeutic Touch really does work? I came up with no single answer, but a combination of all of the above. I finally refused to put a value judgement on it; that was my answer.

Nevertheless, my softly spoken words seemed to have a calming effect on her. I gently rubbed her back and positioned her comfortably. *Should I at least attempt an assessment, try some Therapeutic*

Touch, or should I not disrupt the trusting interaction I feel at this time? Perhaps I'll try it when I know her a little better, I say to myself.

The next day I asked to give nursing care to this patient and again my request was granted. There appeared to be no change in her condition and the physician was visibly upset. His concern is evident as I enter the room. He says, "She's in a lot of pain today and it seems to be getting worse." I look at this frail child and notice that the lines of pain and stress are etched even deeper than yesterday. "I will see what I can do for her," I tell him as I approach the patient. I look at her and she tries to give me a smile, *Is now the time?* I think. *Should I approach the subject of Therapeutic Touch? Will she understand? Will she think I've 'lost it?'* One can only ask to find out and I bring the subject of Therapeutic Touch into the conversation.

I see it in her eyes, a look only a teenager possesses. The look that says *I don't believe what I'm hearing, but because you are a nurse and an adult, I'll be polite.* However, I've gained her trust and her eyes now soften. She says, "Is it like those screaming men on TV who put their hands on people's heads?" I answer, "It is somewhat, but I will do no screaming." She is bright enough to be honest and direct. "I don't think it will help," she says, "but go ahead anyhow." I know that she feels confidence in me and knows that I am trying to be helpful.

Yes, I affirm to myself, *I do want to help.* After centering my thoughts, I begin my assessment of her field. She lies quietly. *What,* I ask myself, *am I feeling? Absolutely nothing!* I find my mind wandering. *Stay centered!* I impatiently tell myself. I try to bring back my thoughts to where I am and what I am doing. I feel that I am losing the concentration of the centering process. I go on, but a voice somewhere inside my head tells me that I am not really helping this child. I feel terribly frustrated and I stop. There is no relief of pain, there is no improvement in her condition. *What am I doing?* Therapeutic Touch did not work for me or for the child. In my mind's eye, I refer back to "the book." I recall that with Therapeutic Touch there is supposed to be an increased opportunity for emotional involvements for which the healer must be psychologically prepared. *Wasn't I prepared? Was this too early in my study of Therapeutic Touch to use it on this child? Perhaps I should have studied harder, or attended more workshops, or conferred with Professor Krieger prior to attempting Therapeutic Touch on this child. But I did try,* I firmly tell myself, *and I must put it aside, accept the consequences and learn from the experience.* The young girl smiles; she doesn't feel any different and her eyes tell me it's OK. This gesture helps to intensify our interconnectedness. Our relationship is changing, each of us getting a better understanding of the other. We are quiet for awhile. I sit in the shadows of the room watching her fall asleep. She is getting restless again. I use my hands to position her, to gently stroke her face, and then I quietly begin to do Therapeutic Touch again. I know now that my very presence in the room is therapeutic to her. I know I can help this child now, for as I learn more about myself, so will I be able to learn more of how I can help her. . . .

The child lies quietly in the bed trying to sleep, while I sit in the chair at her bedside. I close my eyes and center myself. It is becoming easier and easier to center, to get to know myself. It takes less time to get beyond the disturbing sounds in the busy intensive care unit. The child's sleep appears more comfortable now. For the first time since she entered the hospital she sleeps peacefully, without twitching, for two uninterrupted hours.

Was it Therapeutic Touch and the transfer of a different energy that allowed her to sleep? Yes, it was, and I do know for the first time that I am comfortable in this way of therapeutically using myself."

A sense of empathy or sympathy, and an urgent desire to help or to heal, can sometimes move emotions so strongly that it is sensed as an actual felt need, as seen in this exerpt from another student's journal:

"Ms. M., an elderly lady, was out of bed in a wheelchair. When I got to her she was in obvious pain and also in need of personal care. Before we transferred her back to bed, the charge nurse went to get a narcotic for her. While we were waiting, I found myself to be acutely aware of a sense of the patient's energy field. It was the "tightness" of it that impressed me . . . I knew I had to do something . . . I had to ease that block, I *had* to help that poor lady release herself from that taut interweave of tension and pain. This experience was extremely 'tangible'; the needs of the patient were easily transmitted to me, my directions were obvious and I knew with a surety that startled me that there was no way I could just give her an injection, pop her in bed, and simply walk away."

INNER CHANGES

What underlies the dynamics of "directions" arising from within "with a surety that startled me?" Maslow's needs theory offers some useful suggestions. It indicates that there are a number of limited basic ("instinctoid") human needs that are both physiological and psychological. Health, he says, is impossible unless these needs are met. Within Maslow's framework, something is considered a need if its deprivation produces illness.[36] Some years later he extended this theory to encompass "metaneeds"—those things that are necessary for healthful growth towards the actualization of the individual's potential as a human being; i.e., self-realization on the path to "becoming fully human."[37] These metaneeds are related to ultimate values which Maslow calls Being-values or B-values. Deprivation of metaneeds leads to metapathologies which he describes as "sickness of the soul."

The persistent quest for meaning in life frequently evokes a spontaneous inner response that can be described as an upwelling desire to help or heal others in distress. If this aspiration penetrates the bounds of personal needs, there may come a moment of ego-transcendence in which the mere "want-to-help" becomes a "need to help." This works a critical shift of identity from one's ego structure to a perception that is more integrative, being centered in the totality of being, the self. It is from this deeper, more discerning perspective that the need-to-heal reaches beyond the confines of one's own nuclear family, and seeks to alleviate the distress of others. Boundaries between self and other seem to be irrelevant and one responds to the drive initiated by this need-to-heal, whether the healing is to oneself, to family, or to others. This shift to a higher-order perception marks a crucial stage of transformation in the healer. Once the self is deeply engaged, the surge of inner commitment arises from a very different realm, a place of highly personalized experiences whose implications may be very difficult to communicate to others, but which thereafter play a central and unifying role in personal life. Upon examination, the need-to-help appears to lie within the category of Maslow's metaneeds, and rests on B-values of compassion and concern for others. It is not surprising, therefore, that those who embark on the healing way find themselves pressed toward a fuller actualization of their humanness. Directions arise from within with an insistent demand, with a "surety that startles."

INTENTIONALITY AND PERSONAL KNOWLEDGE

It is during this period of transformation that another change in values may occur in the healer. It often happens that a person treads the healing way as an expression of will, of personal power over circumstances. There is nothing essentially wrong with this style: man has raised his fist at the sky for millenia. However, the exertion of will by the healer may exclude the healee from decision-making, (a vital ingredient in the healing process itself). It may arouse a sense of dependency on the healer or even fear of the healer. A more patient-oriented stance is achieved when the shift to perception through the self gains focus and clarity. This perspective makes available a dimension of will that is deeper and more spontaneous than the exertion of personal power: the expression of intentionality. Rollo May has termed this attribute "the missing link between the body and the mind."[38] The connotation of intentionality is not only one of power; it presupposes a knowledgeable relationship between the individual and the object of the intended act. This suggests that not only must the will or need-to-help be present, but also that the healer have a plan for setting the healing process in motion. This makes healing a conscious act rather than a gut-level impulsive demonstration of insistence.*

The crucial step in clarifying intentionality depends upon the healer's conceptualization of how to help or heal the client. The various aspects of this assessment may be integrated in several ways: by logical analysis of the known facts of the problem; by hunch, that is, by an impulsive grasp at passing impressions of the situation; by a spontaneous exercise of intuition during a review of the case

---

*It is important to understand the basis of one's own motivations in wanting to help or to heal. An exercise that has proved useful to students learning Therapeutic Touch, "Listening to Oneself: a Tool for Self Awareness," is included in Appendix A for your interest and use.

history; or by a combination of two or more of these. The value of the analysis is dependent upon the extent and accuracy of our knowledge about the patient's condition. The value of the hunch is that sometimes it is right. The value of true intuition is that it may provide otherwise obscure information in a most insightful and creative manner, frequently in a way that is totally unexpected. Is this a touch of sheer magic? An "answer to prayer?" A display of compassionate grace? An expression of the self through a higher-order structure? Intuition remains a mystery, but we do know that its development can be fostered. Silvano Arieti is quite clear on this point:

> Intuition appears as a kind of knowledge that is revealed without preparation, or as an immediate method of obtaining knowledge . . . The reason why the new knowing or under-standing does not seem to have been prepared is that the subject was unaware of the antecedent stages.[39]

The problem is how to facilitate the generation of those internal cues that precede the intuitive instance. The difficulty is that the direct perception of an immediate situation and its implications escapes our ability to rationalize its process. Because it circumvents reason, Jung designated intuition as irrational. Within the Jungian model, among the functions that differentiate his categories of psychological types, intuition is a perceptual process "prompted by the unconscious dimension" which "at the same time produces an unconscious effect in the object."[40] This suggests some kind of mutual informational processing between the intuitive person and "the object," intuition being an essentially interactional process at a deep level of the unconscious. The question is how to get at it, how to encourage its development and engage its oracular genius in our rather mundane personal interest. Perhaps Assagoli's advice is most direct:

> As (intuition) is a normal function of the human psyche, its activation is produced chiefly by eliminating the various obstacles preventing its activity.[41]

Therefore, intuitive understanding is not a process that we "do," but one that we consciously allow to happen; an "effortless effort," to use the Zen phrase.

A strong, reliable intuition is obviously invaluable to the healer working with the complex imponderables of the human condition. However, how can we rely on a fount of personal knowledge whose source is so little understood in our time?

There is one technique for checking reliability in the teaching of Therapeutic Touch. Students in clinical areas of health facilities are asked to do an assessment of newly admitted patients and write down their findings before they read the patient's chart. They then note any correlations between their assessment and the laboratory findings or other evaluative statements, to learn from their mistakes, reaffirm where they have been correct, realize what they may not have taken into consideration, and so on. Thus, they can personally check out their sensitivity empirically and learn to internalize the experience.

In Therapeutic Touch, assessment involves the use of the hands in a sensitive search of the healee's energy field, for indications of energy imbalance. Actually, the received impression is really an extension of the sense of touch as we usually think of it.* Assessment is always done after the healer has centered him/herself, for this induces a state of consciousness that enhances interior experiences, including the realization of personal knowledge. Under the best conditions, this practice serves as a check on the reliability of our intuition, as well as on the accuracy of the assessment. When this is coupled with an effort to recreate the actual experience of the assessment, it is possible to recall our state of consciousness prior to the intuitive flash, or to remember a feeling tone that served as the cue to that state of mind. Therefore, with continued and conscious practice, the healer begins to gain an understanding of the preparatory conditions that precede and facilitate the intuitive state. Tentatively at first, and then more frequently as repeated trials test out the reliability of such "knowledge . . . without preparation," the healer accepts this higher-order structure and puts it to the service of helping others.

Consistent encouragement and simultaneous testing of the use of intuition in the process of healing may stimulate the unfolding of confidence in this higher-order resource of the self. Over time, and after numerous subjective testings, a sense of certitude may intensify such that a healer becomes willing to trust life decisions

---

*For further details, see Appendix A.

to its insistent urgings. Even though the promptings of intuition may seem unreasonable, irrational, or even contrary to custom, they demand recognition because they have proved their validity. This inner 'listening' becomes in time an innate expression of personal lifestyle, of critical importance in times of crisis, when one 'listens' very carefully, as if to a deeply respected friend.

These higher-order resources provoke experiences in interiority that penetrate into the matrices of the everyday lifeway of the individual as he or she gains experience in the healing process. For this reason a personal experience may serve to illustrate the degree

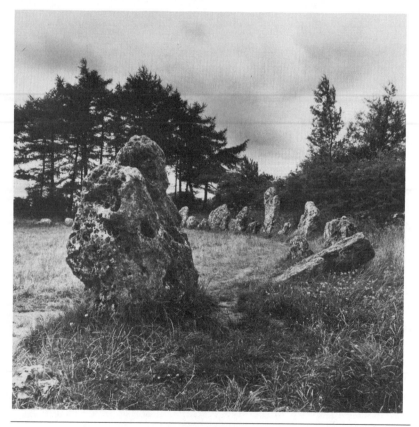

PLATE 1
"The King's Men," a 3,000-year-old stone circle at Rollright
in Oxfordshire, England.

to which one can develop a seemingly unreasonable trust in strong intuitive perceptions. A few years ago, I was invited to London by a private foundation, to present findings on research I had done on Therapeutic Touch, and to teach some of its techniques. The planned schedule permitted me two days to overcome my jet lag, and I was asked how I would like to spend the time. One of my choices was to visit some ancient stone circle other than Stonehenge, which I had heard was quite crowded with tourists. Happily, a friend of the foundation owned a piece of property in Oxfordshire which was the site of another 3,000-year-old stone circle called Rollright. Permission was granted for the foundation's Director of Research and I to visit Rollright and we planned to be there in time for sunrise. Very shortly after our return to London I wrote the following account of our visit, which has been minimally edited or changed in any way.

Sunday   3/14/82

"Ruth picked me up a little after 4 A.M. and without traffic we drove up-country quickly to the private land that is the site for the Rollright stone circle near Oxford. After driving correctly for about an hour and a half, we almost missed it because of an error in, or a misinterpretation of, a final direction. However, Ruth was a very thoughtful companion and gave me both the space and the time to do my own thing until finally the raw, wet cold driven by a penetrating wind forced us to leave and seek out a homey and deliciously warm inn for breakfast. While at Rollright, I felt that I had a quite meaningful experience with the stones and so, with the intention of checking this with knowledgeable friends when I get back to the United States, I decided to record this very subjective impression while it was still fresh in my mind.

"Since the ground was quite muddy, I sat on a low stone directly opposite two comparatively tall stones between which I could see the sun beginning to rise. I suppose the site seemed so good, so vibrant and alive, because the time was close to the vernal equinox. The stones themselves are massive, darkly colored and irregularly shaped, looking rather like large gnomes. They are not straight-sheared as are those at Stonehenge, nor are they of similar material. These stones have many holes in them, seem of volcanic origin, and appear to be deeply rooted in and at one with the earth itself. Wondering how to get in touch with such an ancient structure, I decided to center myself and then allow impressions to arise to consciousness while I meditated.

"The impressions I had were not at all what I think I expected. At one point in my meditation, I became aware of an energetic interchange among the stones, actually between the stones, the earth itself, and the constellations of stars or other bodies then in a particular geometric (astronomical?) relationship to one another. The energy flow was visualized as two distinct styles: one flow concerned itself with the stones themselves and seemed to flow around the circle and through the stones in a continuous cycling of energy. The second flow was quite different; for one thing its flow was linear rather than circular, so that it formed a grid or latticework as it flowed across the circle in east-west, north-south directions. These linear flows formed geometric patterns of triangles, squares, and/or rectangles, all of the geometric patterns interconnected and of one piece. The energy flow seemed the color of white gold and the inside spaces of the triangles and rectangles were of a color I'd describe as black, although that is not precisely what I have in mind.

"As I 'watched,' the impression I got was that the patterned energy flow (I'm not quite sure about the circular flow) was a spin-off or a product of a dynamical interaction between the stones, energy coming from the earth itself and certain constellations then in the sky. The stones, I sensed, acted as transducers for the energy streaming down from these constellations and it was then used in some way by the earth. My impression was that elementals (?) / gnomes (?) /the stone-life (?) were involved in this process and the whole transaction was an important part of the life (i.e., 'behavior') of these stones. As (when?) the laying down of this carpeting of geometric energetic patterning completed itself, there seemed to be a slight tremoring that occurred throughout the structure (which, strangely, was more rectangular than circular so that the energetic structure went beyond the actual stone circle itself) and then the whole energetic structure quietly raised itself as one vibrating piece from the ground, a white-gold shimmering latticework, and effortlessly floated directly upwards from the earth's surface into the sky. At some point it rapidly disappeared, but I didn't see it do so. By this time my eyes shot open in startled surprise, but, of course, I didn't see anything then except the as-usual English countryside blowing in the sharp wind and noted that the sun now was beginning to go behind some scud clouds.

"Many associations immediately flooded my mind, but the predominant one concerned a comparison between the geometric patterning I had perceived and descriptions in various religious works of the tesselated floor of energy evoked by Masonic and certain church ceremonies. On the heels of that association came a very clear thought that human ceremonials (with people) would enhance the effect, if they were done in conjunction or in cooperation with this natural enactment. In the meantime (or, perhaps, in the times when no people took part) these natural forces would diligently continue their never-ending ritual.

"As we left the area, this sense of continuance was reinforced by my last glimpse of the stones as the car sped away: the stones, still looking like giant, hulking gnomes, seemed to be deeply engrossed in the production of another latticework of energy. One had a sense of complete concentration on the task at hand which would go on whether or not we or other people were there. I noticed that although I was relaxed in the car, in addition to a good sense of well being, I felt highly alert and very aware. I realized that I felt a sense of accomplishment, a sense that the impressions I had experienced in some way fulfilled the reason for my coming to England in the first place, even though I had not realized that I had had any 'reasons' to begin with!"

Having committed these impressions to a black-on-white statement that I could confirm or reject upon my return to the United States, I put the matter aside and went to a small dinner party. In the rush of subsequent events, I forgot about the incident until two days later. At that time I was greeting guests in a reception line at the Royal Institute of Great Britain in London, having just delivered my paper.

Toward the end of the reception, a young lady approached me, and said, "Knowing that I was coming to hear your paper and that you had visited Rollright the other day, Don asked me to tell you that he'd be especially interested to know your impressions."

Surprised at the directness of her statement, I played for time by asking, "Who is Don?" and then continued somewhat equivocally, "It was really only an impression." Nevertheless, I went on to give her the above account.

When I finished, she said, "Oh, I see that you know of our Dragon Project."

"Dragon Project? What do you mean by Dragon Project?" I asked, not at all sure whether to take her remark seriously.

"Don has been studying the Rollright stone circle for some time and the study has been named The Dragon Project." She said, "I will see that you get a copy of his latest report."

We parted after that and a day or so later. Ruth handed me the promised report. By that time other priorities vied for my attention as I was preparing to return to the United States, and I put the report in my briefcase.

It was about midway on the return flight that I opened my the briefcase and inadvertently came upon the Dragon Project report. Curious, I took it out and flipped through the pages. As I scanned the report, sentence after sentence seemed to leap out at me. I felt the hairs on my head rise and my scalp actually prickled in sympathetic reaction to my surprise. Several statements on the findings of this empritical study seemed to corroborate parts of my subjective intuitive impressions. Now fully intrigued, I returned to the beginning of the Project report, carefully read it in its entirety, and mused on its relationship to my own experience. The following is a summation of this comparison.

The Dragon Project involved a study into "the nature of stone and the possible routes of energy storage and conversion." 'Don' was Dr. G. V. Robins, at that time a Fellow at the University of London and chief coordinator for physical monitoring at the Rollright stone circle site. The basic assumption underlying the study was that at the molecular level the structure of stone is an incomplete silicate lattice that contains a shifting population of electrons that are trapped in imperfections in the lattice or in microcrystalline cavities. These electrons are in continual flux as they escape from the lattice traps and migrate through the stone. Due to this emigration, there is a small, but measurable, drifting potential that probably drifts to earth in a standing stone. Because of this, "the role of stone in any manifestation of earth energy might be in producing electrical phenomena." Such potential current conveyors would only form a minimal fraction of background "noise," so an effort was made to enhance their absorption of suitable electromagnetic energy. Such a suitable radiation is microwave radiation. To rule out distortion in the silicate lattice from trace metal impurities and magnetic field variation coming from local geographical sources, they decided to monitor the transduction of the incident microwaves by the stone lattice to ultrasonic microwaves. They monitored the ultrasonic effects at Rollright stone circle, known as The King's Men, as well as the nearby lone "King Stone" and the adjacent collapsed Dolmen, "The Five Knights." The monitoring also included a wide radius of the surrounding countryside. The reported findings that seemed to dovetail with my own impressions were:

1. The levels of ultrasonic intensity followed a distinct bimodal distribution with the greatest intensity occurring around the time of the equinoxes and the least intensity occurring during the period of the solstices. At the vernal equinox, it was found that the stone circle activity significantly increased, whereas the activity at the King Stone diminished. (The activity of The Five Knights closely followed that of the King Stone on all occasions. It is also interesting to note that my visit to Rollright took place just days prior to the vernal equinox.)

2. There was a significant differential of activity noted inside the circle, between the stones in the circle and on the stones themselves.

3. The complex waveforms of the periodic pulsations of the ultrasonics indicated that the site activity "continued for the same length of time at all parts and finished abruptly on all occasions."

4. There was "a clear and precise cut-off point, usually a few feet outside the circle."

5. On one occasion, the monitor recorded that as the generalized site activity lessened, the pulsing around the ring of stones nevertheless continued "in the narrow corridor of the perimeter" of the stone circle, somewhat similar "to a cyclotron . . . effect."

The implications of the ultrasonic monitoring suggested to the investigators that the stone circle could be considered "a three-dimensional dielectric antenna whose orientation allows maximum energy transduction at the time of the equinoxes." The investigators also put forward two possible uses that those ancient builders, people of the Bronze Age, might have had for the site: the healing effect that is associated with weak electric fields, and the increased grain germination rates which occur within certain ultrasonic frequencies. The possibility that the Rollright stone circle might be a healing site drew my attention because a similar function was once attributed to Stonehenge. In a 12th Century account by Geoffrey of Monmouth, he has Merlin say to King Ambrosius, in reference to Stonehenge, "in these stones is a mystery and a healing virtue against many ailments."[42] Finally, as I came to the end of the report, I was amused that from my own experiences at Rollright, I would have to agree fully with the Dragon Project investigators' concluding remarks. After discussing various possibilities for future research, they conclude: "Of one thing we can be sure, that whatever we generate, we will continue to be surprised by it."

In reviewing the journals of students to whom I've taught Therapeutic Touch over the years, it becomes clear that an increase in intuitive knowledge (personal knowledge fostered by an intimate engagement of the self), does not appear suddenly. Significant changes in evaluative and cognitive processing occur over time. These are coupled with a more focused attention, a more consciously directed thinking process, a concern for the moment, and an ability for increasingly incisive action. There is neither an immediate liason or identification with the higher orders of the self, nor is there an instantaneous reflection in one's personal life. Rather, the experiential knowledge which springs from the healing enactment, the process of making whole, increasingly reinforces the notion that there is indeed a unitive flow between all living beings and that this flow is focussed and integrated by the self.

Once experienced, this realization can be profoundly transformative. Like the yogi whose goal is an awareness that probes the farthest reaches of human consciousness, the enactment of this realization in the life of one committed to healing/helping others is a journey in interiority that touches on every facet of being. For example, the hands are a primary tool in many types of healing, for human gestures spontaneously reflect the flow of consciousness. The therapeutic use of hands is usually through direct contact with the body of the patient, as in massage, acupuncture, shiatsu, etc. However, as the healer becomes more sensitive to the subtle nuances of the human energy systems, she/he begins to realize that it is both possible and feasible to help/heal without body contact. In other words, the ill person's energy field, or surround, can be positively affected by direct therapeutic intervention, without the need of body contact.

As these experiences are tested for a reality base, and we begin to find such healing interventions reliable as well as useful, it becomes clear that "people do not stop at their skins." If this assumption becomes the basis of regular healing practice, it will gradually become generalized by the healer to other situations and may extend itself to all relationships. As human energy fields, we are not separate; we flow through life together. Insights which arise naturally from the conscious grounding of the self in daily activities as well as during the healing act lead one to a broadening conception of this lack of barriers between people. We have proven to ourselves that people "do not stop at their skins" during the healing act. We humans are really not separated by the limitations of physical form, but are, indeed, without separative boundaries of real significance. One is struck by the essential unity among all beings. What is more, one begins to get a hunch that the invisible but ever-present "surround" not only extends our human energy systems into the space of which we are a part, but also is the field through which we relate to one another. We begin to see space not as a place of separation but rather as an avenue connecting people.

These are some of the subtle ways in which the worldview and the lifestyle of the healer undergo a critical shift. This worldview now becomes the perspective through which subsequent life events are perceived and the basis upon which they are evaluated. In effect, it becomes a self-discipline, a self-directed way of life, a yoga for the healing or helping of others.

CHAPTER THREE
A Yoga of Healing

INNATE HEALING OF THE BODY

Unbalance in our muscles we call tension; unbalance in our body energies is called illness. The latter is the majority opinion of healers throughout the world. Over a very long period of time practice based upon this assumption has demonstrated the truth of this assertion more often than allopathic (traditional) medicine has proved the case, for the concept of "viral diseases." In illness, this unbalance seems to occur as a critical shift in energy that acts to hinder the body's innate self-healing ability.

However, there are many powers for self-healing that are intrinsic to each person: the immunosystem in its nearly infallible recognition of foreign agents in the body; the autonomic nervous system, particularly in its instantaneous protective reaction when the body has been exposed to trauma; the endocrine glands, especially their governance of fundamental body functions, such as the role of the thyroid glands in basal metabolism, concerned with the continual process of building up, breaking down and rebuilding afresh of the body's cellular tissues; the thalamus, in its ability to filter out overloads of physiological stimuli that send their messages to the brain; and a still poorly understood innate ability in the individual to psychologically withdraw or dissociate from an intolerable or sick situation, a kind of ability to filter out overloads of emotional stress.

These several avenues for self-healing, many authoritative persons believe, account for the greater proportion of the successes of healers, and healers themselves openly call upon their use in modalities that are derivatives of autosuggestion, such as autogenic training and guided imagery. To help others who are in pain or distress, anything that will lift a little the mantle of suffering should be used, including persuasion, expectation, suggestion and other aspects of the "placebo effect,"[43] a much maligned and misunderstood concept.

There are also several body tissues that normally display a high capacity for regeneration or self-healing: the skin (which is actually considered an organ), bone, liver tissue and peripheral nerves. Knowledgeable healers take advantage of these functions, too, in the interest of those they would help.

HEALING BY OTHERS

Even though the body is, indeed, an "incredible machine," there are times when the efficiency of these resources is weakened or overwhelmed by various physical and psychological events. It is then that the individual needs help from another person who is willing to become a human support system, using his/her own healthy (i.e., well balanced and integrated) energies on behalf of the ill person. It is a strange paradox that the person who is motivated to help or to heal really does not "have" those energies to give. In the words of Eddington, the famous biologist, each of us is nothing but "an eddy in a stream" of molecules in incessant interchange with other molecules. Nevertheless, it is possible to draw on energy which is not "ours" and use it for the well-being of others.

How does this occur? What underlies the power of human intentionality? At this time these remain questions that have no satisfactory answers. At best we can agree that most healthy people are aware of a vital energy overflow, a vibrant sense of well-being. Those that are compassionate want to share this sense of bouyancy and high-level wellness with those who are ill and so they do an "inside maneuver." Here, they change something—a feeling tone, perhaps—within their being in a little-understood manner. Nevertheless, there is consensus that the "inside maneuver" results in felt changes within the healer and he/she now becomes aware of a highly personalized energy interaction with the ill person.

The major characteristic of this event is a sense of energy flow from healer to healee. Interestingly, although this energy flow is yet to be substantiated by controlled measurements, highly reliable reports by healees (the patients) vouch for a sense of transmission of energy during the healing process. Their descriptions of the changes they feel occurring in their bodies during or directly after treatment is consistent. Most often a sense of heat is felt deep within the body tissues. This is followed by a generalized feeling of relaxation and a sense of well-being.[44] Sometimes there is a slight sense of electrical flow or movement just beyond the periphery of the body. Frequently there is relief from pain, and a demonstrable emotional release may accompany any of these changes. But how do we know these really occur?

REPATTERNING OF ENERGY

The reality of healing, in our time, lies in the actual measurement of physiological or psychological effects. However, there is a general acknowledgment that there are aspects of the healing process— subtle effects of fine energies, experientially known to other cultures as prana, chi, mana, etc.—that are not measurable by the standardized tests thus far designed. These subtle aspects of healing, therefore, remain in the realm of personal knowledge, unrecognized by Western science, even though there is agreement among healers in reports hoary with time.

I can relate an experience which occurred while I was assessing the field of a very young lady who recently had been diagnosed as having a brain tumor. At the time, she was in the midst of a series of treatments from a "psychic surgeon" from the Philippines who was visiting the United States. Although I had never had personal contact with the man, I did not feel it wise to interfere with what he was doing. Therefore I did not attempt to treat her. However, I did agree to assess her energy field. Whatever preconceptions I may have had were quickly dispelled, for as soon as I began the assessment in the area overlying her head I realized there was something in that part of her field which was not at all evident in other areas of her field. To my surprise my hand chakras picked up a gentle but active, rhythmic, controlled, and localized pulsation over a section of one hemisphere. My impression was that these were effects of the healing of tissues then in process, but I doubted then, and doubt now, that there is at this time any measuring machine that can pick up what that human machine recorded.

How can one person so specifically intervene in the repatterning of another's energies? It would appear that control of one's own energies is essential. Perhaps this is so, for healers agree that the first step in true healing is the healing of self, which one could interpret as self mastery. Deep understanding of one's own energies then provide insight into how one can help others.

REPATTERNING OF PERCEPTIONS

From my own experience I have come to think of the process of learning to be a healer—the conscious assistance of others toward a life-affirmative integration of their energies—as an experience in interiority, a kind of yoga, a yoga of healing. Like yoga, the study of healing requires self discipline, it demands a conscious commitment, and it entails a ready willingness to strive towards an understanding of the self-to-self interface, in this case the interface between healer and healee. As such it is an experience at the transpersonal level, a state that harbors possibilities of awareness of the more profound reaches of human consciousness where enhanced perceptions may radically alter one's sense of reality.

Among the characteristics of the healing way are a sense of timelessness during the healing act, an unawareness of the environment or a sense of oneness with it. And yet, there is also a more focused attention, an increase in intuitive processing, a concern for the moment, and a deep resolve towards incisive action. These are hallmarks indicative of significant psychodynamic reorientation regulated by the higher orders of self, which strive towards integration, order, wholeness and self-transformation. Evidence of such high-order emergence can be demonstrated by critical shifts in one's perception and sense of identity, emotional state and evaluative and cognitive processes, in temporal and spatial orientation, and in how one gets meaning from experience. In the practice of Therapeutic Touch, these perceptual patterns are so consistent over time that a measuring tool, the Subjective Evaluation of Therapeutic Touch Survey (SETTS), has been devised and standardized by Fry and Krieger and will be discussed later in more detail. (See pp. 160, 177)

Just how our perceptions transform remains somewhat of a mystery. However, Eliade[45] and others have remarked on the little understood, although long noted, relationship between the spirit and pragmatic experience. It has seemed to me vis-a-vis the healing experience that it is the field or nexus of forces of the unconscious related to both healer and healee which acts as the ground against which these figures of perception interplay. The unconscious is little understood in Western culture, but it is thought to be the catchment of the earliest human experience. In some as-yet-undetermined manner, the dynamics arising from the unconscious are known to influence the individual's thoughts, emotions and actions in daily living.

It would seem, also, that perceptions relate to the individual's perspective or orientation to life. Over thirty years ago Andras Angyal called attention to two fundamentally different patterns of personality, and they continue to be consistent with contemporary thinking. In the first pattern the individual's attention is focused on the assertion and expansion of his self-determination. He feels himself to be "a free, self assertive, striving, autonomous being who organizes the universe around his self," and perceives all relationships within that perspective. The orientation of the second patterning of personality factors is substantively different. This individual's drive is towards becoming an intrinsic part of something greater than him- or herself. This conception is imaged within the context of cultural background and personal understanding.[46]

The healer motivated by compassion falls into the latter category. The healer is a 'channel' or a 'conduit' for the healing energy that might help ill people. Also, it is this self image that may open the healer to a way of yoga as the healing experience deepens and becomes tinged by "the certainty of direct experience" which also defines yoga practice. Naranjo compares the experience of healing to mystical union. He contends that they may in fact be ". . . just different stages in a single change-process."[47]

HEALING AS YOGA

The term yoga derives from the Sanskrit root *yui*: to bind together, or to hold fast (as a yoke). It suggests the bonding of ego and Self, for what is sought by the yogi is the integration of the farther reaches of consciousness with the deeper facets of unconscious. The point of entry for the healer is through the act of centering, for the quietude and serenity that well up from the centering process provide a place of sanctuary for a liason of the restless, questing personality with the imperturbable Self, that nexus of personal knowledge at the hub of one's being. But how does one know that this experience of the mind is real? One must, of course, look to context first.

In the West the definition of reality is objective, empirical and theoretical, in the East this search for reality is subjective, based on self observation and direct experience. Although the empirical methodologies of the West are barely 400 years old (perhaps fifteen generations of transmitted knowledge at most), in the East the modeling upon which the conception of reality is based goes back in a formal manner to Patanjali, circa 200 B.C., who wrote the first systematic description of yoga. This compendium, *Yoga Sutras of Patanjali* (5th ed, Brother Life Inc., 1982), moreover, has high validity and reliability for today. The modern student of yoga who adheres to the path delineated by Patanjali will achieve the goal of union in the same manner, adhering to the same principles as did his or her counterpart twenty-two centuries ago.

Yoga is very often associated with Buddhism; however, it considerably precedes Buddhism. Buddha himself practiced yoga. Patanjali based his systematization of yoga philosophy on the Samkhya system, one of six systems of Indian philosophy. Samkhya is a dualistic philosophy in that it is based on the assumption that the universe evolves out of the incessant interplay and interpenetration of the principle of consciousness, and the primordial substance which underlies all physical form. Within this context, yoga is a method of facilitating and accelerating the evolutionary development of the individual. This is done through self discipline, self responsibility and a self realization based upon the certainty of direct experience. This quest is rooted in specific ethical values, compassion and respect for life. It acknowledges that reality is not above or beyond the daily activities of living, but in the process itself. The purpose of yoga is to identify with the innate structure of one's inner being, the Self. Therefore the yogi turns his or her attention away from knee-jerk reactions to life and living in a recognition that the world is but a psychological projection of the individual.

It is said that the secret of yoga is experience, for the teachings of yoga make use of a language or metaphor that cannot be understood except within the context of experience.[48] Teachings on yoga do not claim to be revelations. They are based on normal human energetic processes whose possibilities have lain dormant due to ignorance about certain universal laws which govern their use. There is little general awareness of these possibilities. The healer, who deals very frequently with these human energies, may acquire access to similar experiential knowledge about the principles that underlie the energetic processes. The grounds for the outworkings of human energy are foci in the human energy field, itself a complex of many interpenetrating fields whose properties dynamically interrelate in a pattern we recognize as human nature. This field functions like a transformer. These foci convert energy systems, or prana, into the kind of energies that make our psychophysiological being what it is. The foci or transformers themselves are chakras. Their primary functions are to collect, change and distribute the prana to the organs of our physical bodies. These foci form the matrix of the chemicophysical field and the psychodynamic field in the individual and set the stage for psychosomatic functioning.

Knowledge of the dynamism of these chakras and conscious experience of their physical functioning through pranic flow is of critical importance to the yogi. Indeed, Govinda, an authority on Tibetan yoga, emphasizes that the physical body is "the sacred stage of an unfathomably deep mystery play."[49] Conscious effort is therefore directed towards plunging the depths of this mystery by using the physical body as test object or probe. The body is made increasingly sensitive to pranic flow by the intense study of the effortless rhythmic nature of the respiratory process through specified breathing exercises. Because yoga must be directly experienced for realization of the different states of consciousness, it lends itself to experimental verification. Knowledge must be pragmatically translated by the yogi into his or her daily acts of living. Transformative changes in lifestyle and in worldview may follow.[50]

Since time immemorial yoga practice has passed directly from master teacher to student. Under close supervision the yogi is offered physical, emotional and conceptual experiences through which she or he may become increasingly aware of the energetic, i.e., pranic, patterns of Self. One must attune oneself to the more subtle frequencies of these energies and bring a clear understanding of their nuances into conscious awareness. To achieve this, one is taught to use the memory of the experience itself as a lead or thread to find the way through the labyrinth of personal events to the source of the experience. The individual then learns to identify very closely with the specific, characteristic energy flows of these experiences. It is in these acts of close identification that the yogi learns to have a conscious, experiential knowledge of how these conduits of prana operate in everyday life.

The ultimate goal is self-mastery in all experience. Taimini describes this personal search as an "intense subjective, supernormal investigation" during which it is found that "all matter, thought and emotion have a subtle media [sic] through which they function." We in the West would call this "vibration." This vibratory interplay of different energy systems demonstrates cohesion and the systems are found to be connected to one another ultimately. According to Taimini, these vibrations can be subjectively followed from one stage to another within the personal experience. They terminate in one fundamental vibratory form or experience which is the source of these vibratory systems. He cites *The Yoga Sutras of Patanjali* for hints on how this can be done.[51]

Healers seem to have an analogous experience when they are trying to determine how to direct their energies to heal another person. Descriptions vary, but it seems that in assessing the healee's state of health, the healer strives for an understanding of the healee's condition by sensing the experiential quality or feeling tone of the healee's energies. The healer then uses this perception as a model. The healer then tries to shape her or his own energies in a manner that emulates or identifies with that model. Many people do this quite naturally in other than healing situations when they deeply empathize with another's emotional states (which are, of course, a form of human energy). On the other hand, when the healer moves on to heal the patient, the model is reversed. The healer now uses her or his own healthy energetic state as the model and tries to reproduce that feeling tone in the quality of energies projected to the healee. Krippner and Villoldo state the case clearly in their discussion of the issue: How can a healer diagnose an illness without knowing a great deal about anatomy and physiology? Assuming that a healer can conceivably employ the full conscious data rate of 10^8 bits of information per second (estimate for certain states of consciousness), they say:

> Perhaps the healer in an altered state focuses on his or her knowledge of one's own molecular structure, projects this onto the healee, and compares it with the more familiar data of

one's own anatomy and physiology, until the disease is diagnosed.[52]

The healer's and healee's energy systems are in a state of close identification. An explicit and graphic description of the healer's experience by the world-famous English healer, Harry Edwards, underlines Taimini's assertion that human energies can be subjectively followed from one stage to another:

> Secondly, with the unlocking of the joints fixed, say, through arthritis or some other cause, the movement of the bones is inwardly felt by the healer. It is a curious sensation as if the movement is taking place within the healer's mind, and by this feeling he knows how far he may go at any one healing session.[53]

SIMILARITIES OF YOGA AND HEALING

It is this certainty of direct experience that forges a very close bond between the yogi and the healer. As with yoga, the deep understanding of healing comes through the experience of the healing act itself. Like yoga, healing as a lifestyle is a *darsana* (Sanskrit): a point of view or comprehension or a vision. In the process of healing others the individual healer can perceive the behavior of the Self reflected in the healing process, and through this interaction the healer understands, or at least acknowledges, farther reaches of his or her own conscious being. It is this perspective of human potential that guides his or her future lifeway.

The medium in which both yogi and healer operate is the incessant upwelling of pranic flow which is individually tailored to each person through her or his chakras. This pranic flow makes itself known through its masterly organization of the cyclic life forces. These life forces are foundational to the life process and are perceived through physical principles that underlie bodily movement, change and transformation. The pranic flow also affects the more human aspects of our being by way of states of consciousness we know as attitudes, behaviors and awarenesses. Human beings are matrices of energetic flows from the heaviest matter of their bodies, i.e., bones, to the lightest of thoughts.

What is it that patterns these diverse flows? In the East there is a concept analogous to Western ideas about lines of force in an electric field or a magnetic field. For instance, iron filings subjected to a magnetic field will pattern themselves along the Hertzian lines of magnetic force. They line up in reference to the positive and negative poles of the magnetic field and define the direction of electron flow. In the East it is said that there are patterned lines of force (*nadis*, from the Sanskrit root *nad*, movement) that carry the pranic flow within each individual being. The worldview one perceives in this modeling, then, is of infinite energies interpenetrating the biosphere. They are cycled in biorhythms, flowing in tides, patterned in force fields, and vitalized by prana, whose organizational base is directed by conscious mind fulfilling its innate directive towards self-awareness.

This is also the worldview of the healer. Regardless of the names these factors are given, the overall schema relates closely to the experience of the healing act. Jung emphasizes this in discussing the chakra system in relation to the psyche: "We are studying not just consciousness, but the totality of the psyche . . . [The chakra systems] . . . are intuitions about the psyche as a whole, about its various conditions and possibilities."[54] Because an understanding of the psychosomatic domain is so central to the comprehension of healing, it is useful to examine more closely some major tenets of this yogic point of view.

YOGIC PERSPECTIVE OF THE PSYCHODYNAMIC FIELD

The classic literature on yoga describes the psychodynamic field in considerable detail. Arthur Avalon, the first person to write authoritative literature on the subject in English, states that the definitive work on kundalini and the yoga practices affected by it was written by a Brahman, Purnananda, in the 16th century.[55] Kundalini is believed to be related to forces deep within the earth, to the cohesive power of matter, to inertia and to the sensation of smell. It is said to be the foundation for the present evolutionary thrust on our planet.[56,57]

There are seven major chakras said to be operative at this time in human evolution (Figure 1), which are descriptively named in Sanskrit. All of them are non-physical, that is, they are foci of force

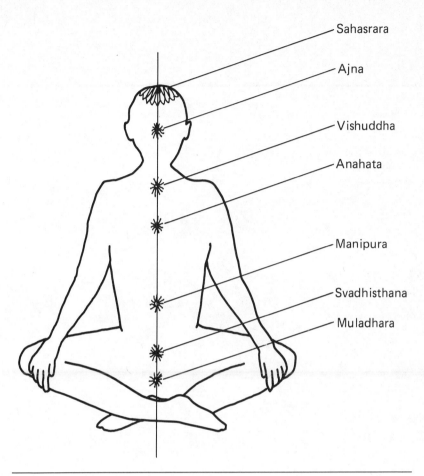

FIGURE 1
Functional centers of the seven primary chakras.

within the human field, and only the lower five are bound in time-space. It was C. G. Jung who first brought them to the attention of Western psychiatry; however, authoritative Western literature on the dynamics of the chakras remains sparse. Swami Ajaya has developed a comprehensive psychotherapeutic paradigm based on insights from the teaching of yoga and extending Jung's ideas on this subject. Swami Ajaya, a student of Swami Rama and a noted psychotherapist, offers a broad classification system of the chakras in cross reference to archetypal themes.[58] He believes that emotional conflicts are due to identification and absorption in the emotional

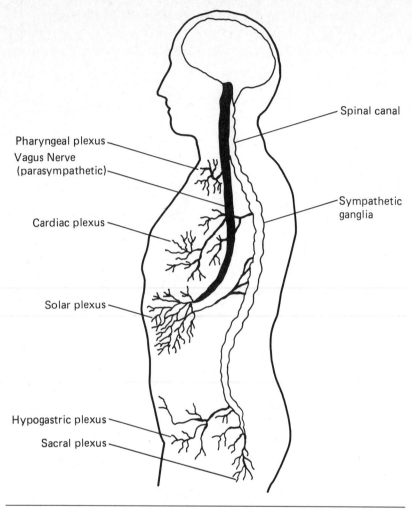

Spinal canal

Pharyngeal plexus

Vagus Nerve
(parasympathetic)

Sympathetic
ganglia

Cardiac plexus

Solar plexus

Hypogastric plexus

Sacral plexus

FIGURE 2
Nerve plexes related to the seven primary chakras.

dynamism of a particular chakra. These conflicts can be transcended, he theorizes, if the therapist helps the client to evolve to the consciousness of a higher chakra (of finer energy). The underlying assumption is that the higher chakras are of a more supportive nature to the indwelling self and mold a progressively more integrated mode of consciousness. Considering the spinal column as a longitudinal axis, the chakras that overlie the spinal cord near the head are said to be the higher chakras, while those lower in the trunk are referred to as the lower chakras.

Overlying the base of the spine is the muladhara (*mula*, root) chakra. Swami Ajaya depicts it as involved with the struggle for survival. He assigns to it the archetypal theme of The Victim. The classical literature says that it is here that the above-noted primal energy, kundalini, remains in a latent state in such manner as to block access to the major pranic circuit, or nadi, called *sushumna*. Sushumna is described as running up a lumen, which is hollowed through the center of the spinal cord, like "a thread through the eye of a needle." Avalon reports it to be the remnant of the hollow tube from which the spinal cord and the brain developed. Sushumna is accompanied by a pair of nadis, *ida* and *pingala*, which are related to lunar and solar energies respectively. These spiral upwards in opposite directions, entwining sushumna as they ascend the field counterpart of the spinal cord, and finally joining with sushumna in a "triple knot" at the site of the ajna chakra, commonly called "the third eye," described below. The three nadis then exit the human field through the field counterpart of the nostrils.

It is said that ascending from the base of the spine to the top of the head there is an increasing differentiation in the vibratory rate and in the functioning of the chakras. These result in more subtle awarenesses being brought into consciousness as one gains successive control of the higher chakras. Motoyama has pointed out that Indian yoga practices for awakening the chakras have a distinctive pattern. The yogi first does specified breathing exercises (*pranayamas*, Sanskrit) to stimulate pranic flow throughout her or his field. Then the chakras themselves are stimulated by the use of certain body and hand postures (in Sanskrit, *asanas* and *mudras*). Finally, through an act of concentration and active imaging, the pranic flow is directed in a manner that activates the chakras.[59] The traditional mode of awakening the chakras has been through direct oral teaching by master teacher to student; however, it is known that there are three points of entry for this learning to occur. These are called the psychic gates. The point of entry is via the coccyx (which probably refers to the muladhara chakra noted above) between the kidneys (the solar plexus chakra?) and at the back of the head, which refers to the throat chakra. Both of these sites are detailed below.

Above the muladhara and at the root of the genitals near the hypogastric plexus of nerves is the site of the *svadhisthana* chakra.

One finds its physical site by marking off four fingerwidths on oneself from the base of the umbilicus. Its functions are concerned with the body's organs of secretion and reproduction. It is a focus for sensory pleasures. Swami Ajaya assigns to it the archetypal theme of The Hedonist. In some systems of yoga its generative functions and its control of the genito-urinary system are considered to be combined with that of the next highest, the *manipura* chakra.

Karlfried Durckheim, a philosopher and psychotherapist, refers to the Japanese interpretation of this chakra. In the Japanese it is called *hara*, literally meaning belly. It is considered to be the physical center of gravity of the body and encompasses the vital center in man. When one puts one's consciousness in hara, Durckheim says, the appearance of the person is of one who is firmly grounded in a deep inner collectedness "from which it receives its force, direction and measure" and "when this center functions rightly, the whole impression is one of evident harmony with inner life." The person who has realized hara and has integrated it into daily actions, learns what she or he is as a living being. In this understanding she or he ". . . can be prepared for anything and everything, even for death, and keep calm in any situation. He can even bow to the victor without loss of dignity and he can wait. He does not resist the turning of the wheel of fate, but calmly abides his time."[60]

Motoyama says that from his experience many sensitive persons who have inherent abilities in psychokinesis (the ability to move objects without making physical contact with them) and extrasensory perceptions appear to him ". . . to have more or less awakened svadhisthana chakra."[61] One school of thought holds that the basis of healing lies in psychokinesis, the ability to move objects at a distance.[62] Nevertheless, Leadbeater, in his modern classic on the chakras, cautions against the deliberate awakening of this chakra, stating that there are very considerable dangers connected with its arousal. In its stead he describes a chakra overlying the spleen. Leadbeater states that this splenic chakra acts as the transformative agent for the subdivision and specialization of prana. Prana is a complex of seven solar energies which break down at the splenic chakra into component parts in such manner that they flow in five main streams to vitalize the body.[63] The functioning of the splenic chakra is disturbed by fatigue, sickness, and extreme old age. From the perspective of Western physiology, the major work of the spleen is directed to the regeneration of red blood cells. It is the function of the hemoglobin component of the red blood cells to distribute oxygen molecules incoming through the lungs during respiration, a constant necessity since human metabolism is mainly oxidative and, therefore, in continual need of fresh supplies of oxygen. In the Indian literature oxygen is said to be a prime conveyor of prana, and so the functions assigned to the splenic chakra seem rational from a Western point of view.

The next chakra of increasing finer energy is called the *manipura* or *nabhisthana* (*nabhi*, "umbilicus") chakra. Its locus is above the umbilicus in the region of the solar plexus. It is said to affect the adrenal glands. It is probably the second of the three psychic gates mentioned above. (The adrenal glands overlie the upper part of the kidneys.) Its functions concern the digestive processes of the body. It is also related to menstrual flow, to breath, to sight, and to the transmission of organic substances into the psychic energies of the lower, more sensuous emotions. It is located in the region of many psychosomatic symptoms which result from pent-up anger, over-whelming anxieties, or deep fear over long periods of time. Ajaya attributes to it domination, competition, a sense of inferiority and pride, and assigns the archetypal theme of The Hero to those who are working out the complexities of this chakra.

Overlying the apex of the heart is the *anahata* chakra. It is concerned with the sympathetic nervous system, the heart, the circulatory system and respiration. It is related to the sense of touch, to the motor nerves, and to the blood system. Its energies are concerned with selfless love, sacrifice and compassion. In Swami Ajaya's archetypal classification, the ideal representation enacted at the anahata chakra is The Savior.

The next progression in state of consciousness is concerned with the *vishuddha* chakra overlying the base of the throat, in the region of the larygeal and pharyngeal nerve plexes. This chakra is the stage for the enactment of devotion, surrender and trust, for creativity and insight, and it is related to breathing and to sound. The vishuddha chakra is considered to be the site of the conscious transformation of prana through mantric power, the power of controlled sound. It is veshuddha chakra that is the third of the three psychic gates noted above. Ajaya finds for the working through of this chakra the archetypal theme of The Child in all its grace and majesty.

The vishuddha chakra is said to be the last site that has a time-space reference. The next two chakras are bound together in a little understood manner and have a different reference frame altogether. The lower of this pair is the *ajna* chakra (*ajna*, command or order) which overlies a region midway between the two eyebrows at the cavernous nerve plexus. It is the seat of both cognitive and subtle senses that lead to insight. It is concerned with the pituitary gland, the autonomic nervous system and the endocrines. The ajna chakra, as noted above, is the meeting place of the ida and pingala nadis which represent the lunar and solar energies. Ajaya assigns to the ajna chakra the archetypal theme of The Sage.

The highest chakra, and usually the last to be fully awakened, is the *sahasrara* chakra, which overlies the top of the head. It is represented as a thousand-petaled lotus (*sahasra*, thousand) and is the goal towards which the aroused drive of kundalini directs itself. It is also associated with the pineal-pituitary axis and is concerned with acts of volition, will (intentionality), altruism, and with states of unitary consciousness. Ajaya does not assign an archetypal theme to this transcendent function, noting that it is beyond form. Archetypes, of course, are not entities in themselves, but represent convergences of behaviors that define an individual as human. Archetypes represent innate predispositions in the individual to organize experience in a particular fashion. They are expressed in image and symbol, allegory and metaphor, and, in our earliest grasp at human-to-human communication, in fable and fairy story.

DESCRIPTIVES OF THE HEALING PROCESS

The certainty of direct experience that arises out of the healing act can be described by a healer in terms of her or his findings about the specific state of an ill person, to another healer of comparable ability. The healer can be understood by another of similar experience and perhaps confirmed in her or his assessment, even though what she or he is describing is non-physical in nature. The modern English language is derived from a technologically oriented culture that still has little understanding of non-conformist modes in which people—instead of a machine or a pill—help or heal other people who are ill. Modern language, therefore, simply does not include within its lexicon words that are fully descriptive of these ancient, but currently little understood, therapeutic human interventions.

I first noted this new word coinage, and new connotations for old words, while I was developing a curriculum proposal for a university course that has its focus on the theory and practice of Therapeutic Touch. My interest was piqued because in Therapeutic Touch much work may be done in the healee's energy field without necessarily making direct contact with his body. I collected these terms into what I called A Glossary of Jargon. However, when I began to analyze them I realized two things: First, the descriptors were consistent among a wide range of healers. Secondly, they readily fell into categories of relevant concepts and impressions that indicated a concurrence of opinion about the dynamics of the human energy field.

In assessing the human energy field most people reported that they could recognize subtle differences in energy states, an energy sense. For instance, a sense of temperature difference was a common experience and could be distinctly labeled as hot or cold. There were several descriptors of the quality of energy flow—a fullness, pressure, tingle, or a slight electric shock. The flow felt stimulated, vigorous, vital, like bubbles or vibes, and these could be either turned on or turned off. In the latter case the energy flow felt as if it were depressed, congested, empty or like a vacuum. Sometimes the flow was sensed as being directional—a magnetic pull towards a particular site or a sense of unbalance in the field. Energy flow also had a sense of rhythm. Its pulsations were orderly (i.e., controlled), in cadence, throbbing, with pattern, without pattern or unstructured, dysrhythmic. The intensity of the flow could be differentiated as strong, weak or attenuated.

It was interesting to find that even in those with moderate experience, during the assessment of the healee's field, emotions could be picked up and correctly identified quite frequently. The terms used to describe them as energy flows were: strong, even, outgoing, good vibes, or ruffled, stressed, taut, restrained, withdrawn, repressed, depressed, or out of control. When healing people who were depressed or whose behaviors were erratic and undisciplined, the healer frequently complained of a sense of depletion of her or his own energies, or a psychophysiological reaction in the healer's own solar plexus chakra.

This finding of a high and consistent level of consensus of descriptions about the healing experience suggests a valid base for a phenomenological approach to the study of healing. Within this reference frame, it would seem plausible that these descriptions might come to be considered valid indicators of a personal process for translating information from one human energy field to another.

USE OF CHAKRAS IN HEALING

There is also strong agreement among healers concerning the different chakras they use under different conditions of healing. Whether the healers have heard about the concept of chakras or not, their experiential descriptions of specific chakras closely agrees with the functions ascribed to them in the traditional literature on yoga practice. For a sensitive healer, as for a committed yogi, these energy foci can become conscious functional centers of awareness, sometimes at very subtle levels. I have found a pragmatic use for this sensitivity, somewhat analogous to Swami Ajaya's psychotherapeutic ploy of first determining the chakra level where the client is presently in conflict, and then helping the client to evolve to the consciousness of a higher chakra from which she/he can achieve a different worldview and so transcend the conflict. In my own scenario, during the assessment of the healee's condition, I gently attune my awareness to my own chakras in an ascending fashion, so that I go into successively deeper states of consciousness. As I do this I simultaneously try to sense whether I can maintain communication with the healee on these levels, i.e., whether a conscious sense of communication exists between us. At some point a limit is reached, which I recognize as either my own circumscribed abilities or the healee's limitations. I then try to maintain this level of conscious communication between our chakras during the healing act.

Other healers tell me that they use one particular chakra, such as the solar plexus chakra or the anahata (heart) chakra, and always project energy to the healee from that specific chakra. Certain Oriental healing techniques (as well as some of the martial arts) make use of the svadhisthana chakra (below the umbilicus) to project *ch'i* (*Qi*). It is by such experiments on oneself that the healer, like the yogi, learns to use her or his chakras with intentionality for the well being of others. This enriches one's appreciation of life and enhances one's knowledge of self and others. It extends into daily activities as the intentional use of the chakras follows easily and naturally.

This experiential knowledge that one can sharpen skills in communication by honing the ability to consciously use the chakras may open other than ordinary levels of communication. Therefore it becomes the responsibility of the individual to exercise intelligent discretion. On first thought this may seem a tricky idea, but that is not the intention. It is now recognized that a basic ability to help or heal others who are ill is a natural potential that can be actualized. These centers of consciousness—which are utterly natural phenomena—can be quickened. As a matter of record, the literature on yoga perceives the successive quickening of the chakras as an expected concomitant of normal processes of human evolution over time.[64]

INCREASED SENSITIVITY

In my own experience I have noticed this concomitant quickening in students as they begin to make Therapeutic Touch a part of their everyday lives. In the process they naturally align and synthesize the functioning of their chakras within the perspective of the higher orders of self. These students become significantly more intuitive, altruistic and articulate. Their thinking becomes noticeably more focused and coherent. Sensitivity to others as well as personal psychic sensitivity deepens. At this time, now that the stigma has been removed from talking to one's plants, it will not seem too extraordinary to learn that many who undergo these changes in awareness feel that they can also communicate with and understand other sentient beings, such as trees, birds, animals, as well human beings. Of course, these persons are the ones who have a green thumb and whom creatures seek out. Another personal story might serve to clarify this ability.

Some people can be quite specific about the chakras they use under particular circumstances. As a child, trees were my first friends. As I got older I felt that I could have meaningful exchanges of thought with them using what I then thought of as different parts of my body, such as my throat. It wasn't until I became deeply involved in the intentional use of chakras in healing, however, that I began to appreciate the specificity of consciousness of the different chakras, and to realize that there is a direct relationship between the species, of trees I communicated with and the chakra that was used.

I thought this was a personal, fanciful notion. A few years ago

I had the distinct joy and privilege of spending some time with one of the most powerful and well-known witchdoctors in Africa, Credo Vusa' Mazulu Mutwa. He is also well known for the quality of his artistic and literary abilities.[65] In discussion we found that we had several experiences in common regarding both healing and the teaching of healing. We discussed the development in persons studying healing of sensitivity to all life forms and the correlation between the chakra one uses in communication with specific tree species. One of my students (they call themselves 'Krieger's Krazies!') taped the conversation, which took place in Soweto, a village outside of Johannesburg, and below is the appropriate section of the transcription. We had been speaking about the effect human emotions have on plants.

> **D:** What I would very much like to ask, sir, is: Do you yourself communicate with plants and trees? Do you find that you are able to communicate with different plants and trees with different parts of your body? For instance, I find that with the trees I live with in northeastern United States, in what the native Americans called the woodlands where most of the trees are hardwood trees, when I communicate with them I find that I do so with this part of me, just beyond or outside the throat.
>
> **C:** Aha! Yes, professor.
>
> **D:** I am very anxious to speak to you of this, sir. In the far West, we have had several very large trees that are many, many years old, the sequoias.
>
> **C:** Yes, the sequoias; I've been there.
>
> **D:** Yes, in the Muir Woods in the Bay Area, for instance. To my surprise, when I am there and I sit and I meditate and I try to get in touch with the sequoias, then I find that I communicate from up here, from the top of my head, from what the Indians call by the Sanskrit term, the sahasrara chakra.
>
> **C:** (*Laughter.*)
>
> **D:** And when I am in the desert and I try to get in touch with the tall cactus—have you been in our deserts in the southwest?
>
> **C:** I was in the Navaho desert.
>
> **D:** Ah! I've been adopted by an Apache-Mohawk native American family. I'll show you a picture of my sister, Oh Shinnah, and the family. But to go on, when I attempt to communicate with the tall cactus then, again to my surprise, I find that I communicate

through here, through the solar plexus chakra, and obviously from the look on your face, you do, too. (*Laughter*.) This is what I would like to share with you.

C: You see, professor, let us say, now I am talking with one of those trees which grow near here. I find there is a slight cold in my feet, around about here in my legs (pointing to certain secondary chakras in the legs). The more deeply we communicate, the more the slight cold rises. The same, exactly the same as you feel. This tree is not indigenous to Africa. We use this (other) tree for the treatment of rheumatism. Now, when I am trying to talk to that one, its spirit comes not to me through the body, but through the top of the head. Now, I thought I was the only one who felt this, but others do too.

As a result of that meeting, Credo had a necklace made which he blessed and gave to me, and he also gave me a name. In Zulu it is *Uyezwa*, which translates as She Who Understands. I look upon

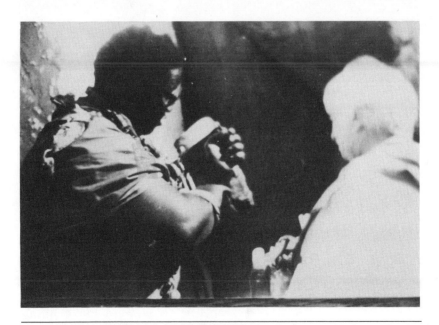

PLATE 2
Credo Vusa' Mazulu Mutwa, well-known African witchdoctor, artist, and author, explaining various symbols on his bronze and malachite crown to the author.

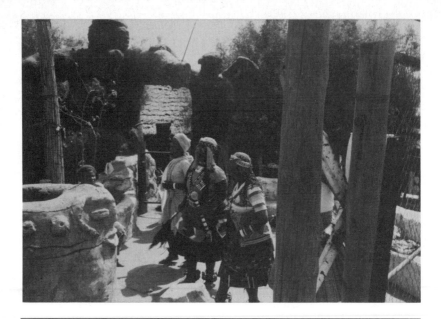

PLATE 3
Students of Credo Vusa′ Mazulu Mutwa dancing.

this name as a kind of credentializing. It stirs within me the realization that these experiences are real, and have a validity to which
others can attest.

Talking to trees (and having them answer!) may seem quite far-
fetched; however, there are many down-to-earth situations in which
one can prove to oneself, if not to others, that there is validity in
intentional exchanges between oneself and nonhuman consciousness. For the healer this sensitivity is not an end in itself, but arises
as a natural concomitant of increased sensitivity to all that is living.
Another personal incident is still very vivid in my own mind, even
though several years have passed. It may serve to demonstrate the
quality of this sensitivity. A friend had flown with a young red setter
dog directly from Paris to Pumpkin Hollow Farm, where the original research and practice of Therapeutic Touch were done. During
the night the dog had been let out and did not return, and so in
the morning the fifty or so people at the Farm formed search parties
to find her. Everybody went off in cars. However, I did not own
a car and so I set off with my own dog to search the meadows and
backwoods.

It was a very hot summer day and after an hour or so of searching I sought out the cool shade of a large, and very old, maple tree. I sat with my back against its trunk and idly watched my dog sniffing out territory. I thought to try to get in touch with the maple tree, and so I centered myself in what I thought was the appropriate chakra to communicate with this tree. I visualized the lost dog as clearly as I could and asked the tree if he knew where I could find her. I was aware of a response within myself almost immediately: In lucid terms it told me to go towards a well-known lake and to ask the people as I went. Somehow this message instilled within me a sense of urgency. I quickly whistled up my dog and took off in the direction of the lake without questioning the instructions.

I cut across the meadows with a sense of purpose until I got to the lake road. I then stopped at every farmhouse on the way to find out whether anyone had seen the dog, since this was my interpretation of the information from the tree. Although I visited every farm along the way, I finally arrived at the lake without turning up a clue to the whereabouts of the dog.

By now it was late in the afternoon, and as I looked at my tired pooch I thought we had been following a will-o'-wisp which had originated as a figment of my own imagination. There was a free-standing telephone booth at the lake shore and I phoned the Farm and asked a friend to drive over to the lake and pick us up. It was then that the miracle happened. As I looked up from the phone, I saw a middle-aged couple, evidently tourists, walking along the lake's shoreline. Remembering the information to ask people as I went to the lake, I went forward (with some ambivalence, I admit) to meet them and ask about the lost dog. Incredulous as it may seem, the wife turned to her husband and said, "Dear, wasn't that a red setter dog that was with the gateman when we drove back to the hotel last night?" The husband agreed and we all walked over the nearby isthmus of land to a hotel situated on a bit of isle in the lake.

The husband sought out the hotel manager, who brought the gateman to us. Yes, he said, the dog we described had come to the gatehouse about 11 P.M. looking as though she had been running. He gave her some cool milk and she stayed with him. About midnight one of the chambermaids was driven back to the hotel by her brother-in-law. They stopped to chat and the conversation turned to the dog. The gateman regretted that he could not keep the dog because of hotel policy and in reply the brother-in-law said, "Well, would you let me have her? We need a dog at the house and we'd give her a good home." The gateman gave the dog to the brother-in-law and they drove off.

That was all the gateman could tell us, but he did seek out the chambermaid at our request. She, in turn, confirmed the story and told us that the dog had been taken to a very large town about 50 miles from where we then were. She gave me her brother-in-law's address and telephone number and—thanks to quite explicit advice from an old maple tree—dog and mistress were soon reunited. For me, this experience gave me the incentive to initiate a continuing series of experiments to test the reliability of extended means of human communication that seem to arise so naturally and so readily in those who seriously turn their attention to seeking out cues about others' states of consciousness during the healing act.

One can look upon this incident from points of view quite different from the one I suggest—the explicit advice of an old maple tree. However, one can learn from these inner experiences. Needleman says, "the real human learning involves an exchange of energies and an interaction of forces identical in nature to the movement of forces by which the universe itself comes into being." One accepts its validity, he says, because the experiences "resonate within the interstices" of the grid of events in one's life.[66] In healing, I would say, much of this meaning comes through the process itself—the experiential, subjective search for personal values and beliefs. The interplay of inner events comes to conscious awareness through the media of metaphor and intuition, subliminal cues and paraconscious cognition, subtle physiological changes and deep "gut" feelings. These are unfettered primal energies that may thrust themselves to the forefront of the too-frequently censored and circumscribed focus of our immediate attention. They force the recognition that we are of a similar nature as the universe.

PSYCHODYNAMIC STRUCTURE OF THE EMOTIONS

There are many more instances of the use of chakras as founts of consciousness in daily life. Chakra dynamics are considered by many cultures to be as natural a factor in human psychophysiological functioning as is the functioning of the autonomic nervous system in Western culture. The prime characteristic of the psychodynamic field is that of a psychic continuum from quite rudimentary sensations to highly sophisticated and complex emotions.

How is this psychodynamic field realized in the world of experience? We in the West are still strongly engaged in the study of human depth psychology and therefore our conceptions about our emotional nature have not yet fully stabilized. From a psychophysiological perspective these feelings are basically responses to sources of pleasure or pain. There are more extended definitions in other cultures, however.

The Hindu conception, for instance, sees each individual consciousness as clothed in successively more compacted living vestments, or "sheaths" (kosha) of matter during what we would call embryological development. At birth and during the subsequent growth and development of the individual, these sheaths are the avenues for the functioning of human consciousness. In a sense the sheaths are somewhat analogous to the construct of energy field in Western science and, therefore their characteristics might be thought of as human energy field phenomena. Within the Eastern frame of reference, the initial focus of attention is at the level of the unitive link with that formless consciousness that has been given a multitude of names and yet is indescribable: The Void, the Source, the All, the Great Spirit, etc. The Hindu name is *anandamayakosha*. Loosely translated, it is the sheath (kosha) of illusion (maya) through which bliss (ananda) is perceived.

The next, more physical, domain or sheath of individual consciousness is akin to what we would call the Overself, one's highest archetype, or God. Its functions concern abstract thought, intuition, the ability to conceptualize and discriminate (*vijnanamayakosha*). From there the consciousness preparing itself for physical birth gathers a perceptual apparatus that allows the development of an increasingly focused ego. Over time, the intellect of the growing person is used as a tool for analysis or logical deduction and emotions, which are the basis for the functioning of desire (*manomayakosha*). The physical body itself is vitalized by the *pranamayakosha*, which is concerned with the distribution of prana, the life energy system that underlies the organization and function of the life process in man. The final and most dense sheath (*annamayakosha*) is concerned with the reenergizing of the physical body through time by the digestion and assimilation of food.

These sheaths might be described as life force fields. Within this context, then, one could align the idea of the psychodynamic field, mentioned above, with the concept of the manomayakosha. Through a synthesis of Eastern experiential knowledge and Western empirical research findings, we could broaden our understanding of ourselves as human beings. Consonant with such a context, deeper questions could be asked: How is the psychodynamic field experienced?

At the onset one realizes that there is something basically distinct about this psychodynamic facet of the human personality. It is a fundamentally different energy system than other avenues of expression. It is specifically designed so that the inner reaches of the individual can gain the experience of sensation. This unique field produces, systematizes, and lends subjective bias to thoughts about these sense perceptions. These impressions enable us to feel alive.

There is a characteristic restlessness or constant shifting inherent in this process so that thoughts and emotions are ever-changing. This underlying dynamic exhibits irresistible drive and exposes psychological needs, appetites and passions which may be violent if uncontrolled. This domain of human psychodynamics is intensely alive, sensitive and impressionable to external events. It responds with a full spectrum of feelings and thoughts.

THE CONSCIOUS USE OF THE PSYCHODYNAMIC FIELD

Ancient Eastern teaching on yoga tell us that the psychodynamic field interpenetrates physical matter and, in a sense, occupies the same space. Therefore, it is not a place but a condition of nature. It is said that it exhibits a sevenfold increasing density of matter in which it operates. As an expression of consciousness the psychodynamic field is free and unrestrained in its own domain under certain conditions, such as sleep, coma, out-of-body experiences, near-death experiences, and death itself. In the ancient traditions, textbooks such as *The Tibetan Book of the Dead* and *The Egyptian Book of the Dead* use the process of dying and the death experience as analogies by which the student was taught conscious use in his or her daily life of the laws and principles of the psychodynamic field.

Is there a way that we, in our time, can also learn to understand and use the natural powers of our own inner natures to meet contemporary exigencies? Today stress-related illnesses are pandemic, even in third world countries, and so we all have grave need for the touch of the knowledgeable healer. A constant bombardment of stressors have coarsened our daily reactions to events and to our relationships with others. With the loss of sensitivity we also have lost touch with the vital reciprocity and resiliency of our psychodynamic nature. This dynamic is the source of innate powers that allow us to interact with others and maintain the integrity of our own being. It is a crucial factor that gives us access to self-healing as well as the helping and healing of others. There is, therefore, urgent need to once again recapture this inner connection and reclaim our natural sources of protection against the insidious toll of stress-related dysfunction. For those committed to the helping or healing of others, the binding of one's life-sustaining energy in the service of personal anxiety and fear cannot be accepted. Healers, as well as helpers, need to act *consciously*.

If we look to what the ancients have told us about the psychodynamic field, and couple that with contemporary information and with the personal knowledge we derive from engagement in the healing act, we can catch hints about ways to release our own psychodynamic field energies (manomayakosha) and thereby allow these energies the unencumbered free flow of their own natures. We know that it is characterized by constant restless motion. Therefore, it is highly labile and subject to change. It is sentient, life-striving, and has a very broad expressive range of emotional patterns. It is exquisitely responsive to external events. It has the capability of translating these encounters to the consciousness, which then molds our physical attributes in the image of these reflections.

From contemporary studies, particularly in the psychosocial sciences and from experiences in healing itself, we can infer that strong emotions apparently sweep through the psychodynamic field, setting up relationships with other emotional patterns in their path.*

---

*It may be difficult to imagine the highly mutable nature of energy in this time of formal, staid perceptions. An exercise in visualization developed for this purpose may be of some use. See Appendix B.

We might further surmise that the size of this pliant field correlates strongly with the intensity of the emotion. From studies on psychosomatic effects it is also reasonable to assume that constant or frequent disturbances in the field set up eddies, or centers of dissonance, in energy flow. It can be deduced that this turbulence may result in the dysynchrony of the psychodynamic field patterning that we call emotions. Taking a cue from biophysics, it can be reasoned that such repetitive discordance in the energy flow may overstress the structuring boundary conditions, whatever they may be, and lead to breakdown or attenuation in the integrity of the field. Perhaps it is this violent disruption of pattern that sets the stage for the vitality leakages and the energy imbalances perceived by healers as an invariable accompaniment of illness. We do know from high-tech tests and measurements that such overstress of the emotions act to depress the body's immune response. Depression of this guardian system of the body may open the individual to psychosomatic disorders, diseases of the nervous system, and, perhaps, dysfunctions we have yet to recognize and define.

How can we put this information together in a conscious effort directed toward the well-being of people? To sustain the integrity of this substantial ally in healing, the psychodynamic field, we need to maintain the integrity of its being. The free flow of sentient energies acts to pattern and repattern our emotions in healthy, vivid response to events and relationships within as well as outside our person. We know that strong emotions have a resonating effect on other emotional patterns. By some little-understood sympathetic vibration, other patterns in the psychodynamic field respond to the high energy of potent emotions. They sensitively repattern, reflecting this change. This is the source of the force and power of strong emotions. If these emotions are elevating, we feel lifted up in a sense of well being. Studies have demonstrated that such a state of mind enhances the drive towards high-level wellness.

To use these innate powers with understanding, the healer must act, as does the yogi, from the certainty of direct experience and must apply this knowledge about human energy field dynamics to the conscious use of one's own energies in self-healing and in the healing of other.* For the past four hundred years it has been

---

*For exercises on human energy field dynamics, see Appendices C, D, and E.

precisely the validity of inner experience that has been denied, and in its place reality has been defined solely on the basis of objective empirical findings molded to a mechanistic frame of reference. The present time is witness to a new interest in the comparison and synthesis of ancient knowledges with recent learnings about the basic structure of our universe. Out of this more humanistic perspective has come unprecedented support for inner experience as another way of knowing. It is within the context of this new knowledge that the yoga of healing is finding substantive documentation and validation as an enactment of what is essentially an experience in interiority, and it is the outworking of this experience in interiority that effects shifts in the attitudes and worldview of the healer and, ultimately, acts to change his or her lifestyle.

CHAPTER FOUR

The Healing Act as an Experience in Creativity

*T*he response of living things to the healer's hand, more often than not, is an enigma. Healing, once in progress, seems to take on a life of its own. The need to heal seems to well up from a depth little known to the healer, and to progress with a surety of purpose that can elicit a sense of awe. The healer is as a spectator watching the repatterning of vital energies taking place, forced to realize that there is an intelligent process at work. The healer is little more than a channel, or conduit, for a suprarational ordering process.

In the *Phaedrus*, Plato remarks that healing is one of the direct ways that the divine makes itself known at the physical level.[67] As the contemporary healer witnesses the healing process unfold she or he would acknowledge this, although a different terminology might be used. To the degree that the healer is committed to healing/helping others, a continuing personal quest for sensitively understanding this healing intelligence becomes one's lifeway. This persistent striving to understand an event as part of the order of the universe comes close to Silvano Arieti's definition of creativity,[68] and I have been impressed for many years with the increasing realization that in fact the healing act and the creative act have much in common.

SIMILARITIES OF CREATIVITY AND HEALING

In both creativity and healing there is an irresistible drive to reach beyond one's usual capacities. The creative act may or may not have a deeply motivated base. Much of creativity appears to both creator and observer to be spontaneous and without a specific goal. The highly personalized nature of the healing act is frequently charged with powerful emotions directed outward, away from self, towards the helping of another person. The two act synergistically to help the healer reach beyond the limitations of his or her ego. This lends an altruistic cast to the endeavor that serves to shift the tightly bound egocentric identification. With the loosening of the rigid controls of ego, one's awareness becomes more acute, and perhaps more insightful, as the healer reaches into facets of him- or herself that previously were not consciously recognized. The need-to-help, the compassion that accompanies the healing act, also acts to vitally energize the quest, as does the struggle to translate verbally to others what are essentially nonverbal states of consciousness experienced during the healing act. In the process, the healing act becomes a fundamentally different perception. Its living center is a sustained experience in interiority in which the healer turns his or her attention within towards the innermost reaches of his or her consciousness of self.

CHANGE IN EGO STRUCTURE

Students of depth psychology, which studies the profound powers of the unconscious that are at work on "the hinterlands of the self," say that when there is "a withdrawal of the center of psychic gravity [focused] around the ego . . . [there follows] the creation of a new psychic condition that is not ego-centric but excentric, meaning that the center of consciousness is in a state of flux."[69] This active process of reorienting the specific contents on which the ego relies was called by C. G. Jung the individuation process. It is thought of as a psychodynamic operation regulated by the self that ever strives towards integration, order, wholeness, and self transformation. In the person engaged in the healing act, this high-order emergence of the self is demonstrated by significant shifts in perception and sense of identity, in marked changes in emotional states and evaluative and cognitive processes, in a different sense of temporal and spatial orientation, and alterations in how one gets meaning from experience, as the finer energies of self come into focus.

The healing act itself, usually accompanied by a dramatic quieting of gross psychomotor activity in the healer and frequently coupled to a relaxation response in the healee, produces a milieu that is conducive to creativity. A profound sense of relatedness often envelopes healer and healee, an at-one-ment in which both may have a tacit knowing of the other in a manner that is "more than one can say," to use Polyani's expression.[70] If the healer has consciously centered him- or herself, this experience in interiority may have considerable depth, and an expanded realization can occur of how the healer may help the healee.

EMPATHY AND ENDOCEPTS

Initially this increased awareness often takes place at a preverbal level. This nonverbal and preconscious or unconscious cognition seems to be energized by a strong sense of empathy for the healee. In this diffuse and amorphous state, the condition resembles what Arieti has termed endocepts, primitive organizations of previous experiences, memory traces and images of things and movements that are perceived as felt experiences or gut feelings that cannot be clearly described with words.[71]

Endocepts search for ways to express the inexpressible. Through this intensive press for meaning they may undergo transformation into communicable symbols, images, reveries, etc. Once their content can be communicated, they may act as a basis for creativity via a stunning moment of inspiration or intuition that serves to translate the endocept into a conceptual form which lends itself to expression.

The attitude that the healer takes during this time, which is similar to that assumed by the creative person, is one that I have called "listening," a quiet, focused inner awareness by the healer of any cues of imbalance or dissynchrony, congestion or stasis in the energy systems of the healee.[72] It is a kind of creative listening in which the healer uses all the "antennae," the sensory receptors at her command, to pick up cues that suggest degrees of differences between his or her field dynamics and those of the healee.

NONLOGICAL BASIS FOR ASSESSMENT

Just prior to the assessment of the healee's condition, the healer goes through an incubation period during which bits of information from several different contexts of experience are brought together. Where these data can be integrated and synthesized, new insights into the healee's condition may arise, which the healer then acts upon in the interest of the wellbeing of the healee. This is not necessarily a logical process. In the best of cases, I see an analogy between the healing assessment and the riddle (*koan*) given by the Zen roshi to the student; this riddle is unsolvable, if only the intellect is used. Just as for the Zen student, the intellectual solutions that had served so well in the past won't work in this realm, where energy patterns rather than intellectual constructs are the reality. The modeling of the human energy field assessment in healing is not based on the Greek logic that underlies the traditional medical model, for example, and other disciplines based on empirical reality.

Being thrown upon a nonlogical system serves to produce in the healer a somewhat anxious state, perhaps culminating in an inner crisis. When it is recognized that intellectual skills may not be either useful or appropriate in this type of interaction, the healer may put aside this rational approach and let go. Quieting the chattering monkey—the constant monologue that the waking brain engages with itself—the healer just "listens" to what his or her hands "tell her." To do this the healer sensitizes him- or herself to subtle inner cues, synthesizing and resynthesizing the various bits of information as they come through his or her many sensory pathways. The healer is able to sense the unity underlying the diverse patterns of data. With this shift of figure and ground, the interior experience (rather than the external experience) becomes the reality. The problem may be perceived suddenly in a new way that may be truly insightful.

This creative leap is similar to the resolution by which the Zen student finds the answer to his *koan*. It is very much like the catalytic moment of the creative person's flash of inspiration. There are, of course, several modes of consciousness, each appropriate and valid within its own context or level of reality. The brain, which we often think of as our major avenue of consciousness, offers a variety of methods for processing data. It is also within the capabilities of human consciousness to restructure and transform information to meet contingencies, conceive original ideas or weave outright fantasies out of the mind-stuff of daydream, reverie, recollection, or intuition. Beyond this, there are other functions of consciousness that are differentiated from both the physical body and the mind. They transcend the capabilities usually attributed to human consciousness and therefore constitute a foreign territory of cognition for most of us. Some of these higher-order functions were described in Chapter 3 as being familiar to both yogi and healer. In fact, this level of function is common ground for all those illumined by the intuitive flash of high creativity and inspiration. For the healer, entry is granted through the engagement of the self in an altruistic act of helping/healing another. This can become an experience in the transpersonal. This very different vision of reality can then act as a touchstone for the urge towards the novel and the creative.

THE HEALER'S RESEMBLANCE TO CREATIVE PERSONS

There are several characteristics of the truly creative person[73] that may be shared by the committed healer. From the first felt urges of the need-to-help, the search for the meaning of human suffering is directed inward. In service of this quest, one's own needs and desires are restrained and disciplined to meet the needs of others. The clients of the healers frequently come to them because more conventional avenues of help have not stemmed the tide of illness and its consequences. Frequently the urgency of a last minute surgical operation serves to stimulate and heighten the healee's expectations as well as the healer's efforts. Since the healer's frame of reference is in human energy systems, not the formal classification systems of medical diagnosis, she or he is not restricted by the systematic boundaries of logical analysis. This freedom allows the healer access to a wider variety of experiences and the opportunity to engage in different models of reality. Because of this, the healer may make significant contact with unconscious realms of experience. Much of the effective interaction between healer and healee wells up from the unconscious in subtle ways. Journal entries of my students indicate the dynamics of this process:

"My husband had a bout with bursitis last week and was in considerable pain. I had not told him the details of this course at school because he tends to be very critical and skeptical of anything that appears 'far out,' and so rather than leave myself open to attack, there are several things in my life that I have not shared.

However, his pain was real and unrelieved by medication and finally I decided to approach him with the idea of Therapeutic Touch. To my surprise and delight he shrugged his shoulders and said, "Well, what have I got to lose?" I quickly explained Therapeutic Touch to him and began. I took a moment to center myself and then I assessed his energy field and felt the bonding of love between us. Suddenly, in a timeless moment, new knowledge about my husband of several years seemed to bubble up from psychological depths shared by both of us. I realized then that although he had a deep, unexplainable fear of anything he couldn't see, he trusted me.

He laughed when I began to work on him, but in a few moments he said, 'Hey! What are you doing? My shoulder feels warm.' I had felt an area of density in the field over the left scapula and tried to get the congested area to flow freely again. After about five minutes I could feel a more equal balance of energy on both sides of his field.

My husband was amazed! He hunched up his shoulders and then moved them freely around and around. His face looked relaxed, free of tension and pain, and he acknowledged, "it does feel better," and then turning around to look me full in the face he continued, "You know, you and that occult stuff really used to scare me sometimes!" I felt that there had been a significant breakthrough in our relationship . . . and knew it for sure when, after another timeless moment, we both realized that we were standing in the middle of the room, vacantly smiling at each other like a pair of idiots with a big secret, not touching each other, yet each knowing with a fullness that had neither barriers nor boundaries."

Another similarity between the creative act and the healing act is that the healer is able to integrate inner experiences with the conscious mind and bring forth new patterns of expression, new ideas. One of the memories I have of unique, creative healing under seemingly impossible circumstances concerns Delia, an Eskimo doctor that I met in Kotzebue, above the Arctic Circle in Alaska. The United States Public Health Service sent me to Alaska at that time to teach health officers Therapeutic Touch with the thought that it would act as a liaison between the more formal medical world of the public health officers and the world of the folk medicine of the native Eskimo doctors. Upon my arrival in Kotzebue, the public health hospital gave a party for me, and Delia was one of the guests.

It took very little time for Delia and I to get into a deep conversation comparing our experiences with different healing techniques. Delia is particularly known for her innovative methods for delivering babies born under difficult or unusual conditions. She shared with me her technique for safely delivering babies that are born with the umbilical cord twisted around the neck. This technique, which she developed while living out on the tundra, is highly creative and elegantly simple.

The technique is based on the fact that the unborn child is surrounded in utero by a watery medium, the amniotic fluid. Delia sits facing the pregnant mother, directly in front of her abdomen. She then extends her arms on either side of the abdomen so that the inner aspects of her wrists are about one inch from the abdomen. She then rhythmically flicks her wrists inwardly so that they repeatedly tap on the tautly stretched skin at the sides of the mother's abdomen. Delia explained that the "pumping" puts the amniotic fluid into motion "like little lapping waves." This rhythmical ebb and flow of the watery medium, she said, serves to float the umbilical cord and loosen its hold around the baby's neck. Delia uses her sensitive fingers to gently palpate the mother's distended abdomen, feeling for the beat of the unborn baby's umbilical arteries to determine when the baby is free of the entwining umbilical cord. The heroic high-tech measures resorted to by professional persons under similar circumstances, and the sense of helplessness of those in primitive conditions equivalent to Delia's, suggests that the elegant simplicity of her method for freeing the babe from the strangulating umbilical cord is also profound.

Healers in the creative mode have a willingness to experience emotion in themselves and in their patients, and bring to these experiences a sensitively attuned awareness. The importance of rapport between healer or therapist and patient has been noted in many cultures. It was the foundation for Sigmund Freud's recognition of the use of transference as a powerful therapeutic tool. Frequently the first clue that the patient has that he or she is permitted to relate emotions to the therapist or healer is as a spontaneous response to the felt quality of the healer's approach. During the healing act rapid strides can be made in this permissive atmosphere to get at crucial psychological features underlying the illness.

The creative healer also has the ability to accept ambiguity, to seek out new frontiers of performance and not be bound by pre-formed ideas. A student relates a fairly good example of this occurrence while at work:

"Mr. E. T. was an eighty-three year old patient who had a craniotomy for the removal of a subdural blood clot which he had sustained when he fell on the way to his office. The daily clinical report stated that he had been having periods of confusion and restlessness, but the medical opinion was not to use sedatives on him since they might mask his mental status and level of consciousness.

"I was on night duty when Mr. E. T. became extremely agitated and seemed disoriented. He had an expressive aphasia,* and his difficulty in the use of words made it almost impossible for the nurses to readily determine what was bothering him. His bed was not directly observable from the nurses' station and he didn't have a roommate to watch him. When he attempted to climb over the bedrail, cloth restraints were applied to keep him from falling; however, they were applied with considerable hesitation since he had a history of inferior wall myocardial infarct.*

"Mr. E. T. became increasingly agitated and tried to free himself from the restraints around his chest. We seemed to be helpless to prevent this man from harming himself. Suddenly I thought of Therapeutic Touch, but seeing the man so violently thrashing around his bed I was very skeptical that Therapeutic Touch would work and I hesitated. However, as I watched Mr. E. T. throw himself about and realized his feelings of exaspiration and frustration, I was moved beyond my own concerns. Nothing else seemed to work and nobody else seemed to be willing to help; I felt impelled to try.

I began by centering myself with the intent of searching out some inner guidance for a way to help this old man. In my assessment I felt considerable heat over his head. He probably has a headache, I thought, but I nevertheless focused on that clue and worked on him without noticing the passage of time or being aware of the background noises in the corridor. The patient began to relax and

I soon noticed that he closed his eyes. By the time I finished the treatment he was fast asleep.

He was lying on his right side when I left him to take care of other patients. I checked him about a half hour later and he was still in the same position, fast asleep. Three and a half hours passed in this way, the patient still assuming the same position, his relaxed posture and quiet, even breathing assuring me that he still slept. In the morning, however, he was easily roused. His eyes appeared clearer and brighter and he looked calm and rested. He smiled when I greeted him, took his medications and went back to sleep."

ENCOURAGING CREATIVITY

It was Carl Rogers who pointed out that we cannot expect an accurate description of the creative act, except in a general way, because by definition its very nature is indescribable.[74] However, we do know that the inner processes that prepare the ground for creativity can be fostered. As noted earlier, it is my impression that there is an apparent close fit of the significant characteristics of the creative act and of the healing act, both of which are based in a high-order emergence of the self. How, one wonders, can such unique ability be cultivated? Certain pragmatic factors have been reported. Of prime importance seems to be the establishment of an atmosphere in which conditions for creativity are permitted and encouraged to emerge. Such an atmosphere would be non-judgmental and would be designed to assist the individual to express and to actualize his or her potential in novel and spontaneous ways. Not only would the individuals in such a milieu be accepted, an empathic understanding of each for the other would be actively supported. In this way a climate would develop that permitted the free expression in each one of the deepest reaches of the self. Mature societies in the past have recognized, honored and emulated their creative members. Perhaps in the future society will recognize that a similar inner experience awaits those who espouse what is one of the most humane of human acts, the helping or healing of others and actively, and creatively, support those who would lend themselves to this life-affirmative lifestyle.

Reflections on Therapeutic Touch

I have reached for you in many ways
one of which was to run
at speeds so fast
I seemed to stand still
while you danced around me.
Now, caressing invisible forces
passing through your field,
I've discovered the tempo
and dance to your beauty
which is mine.

L. Mowad, M.A., R.N.,
A Krieger's Krazie

CHAPTER FIVE

Therapeutic Use of the Paranormal

A BASIS FOR PERSONAL KNOWLEDGE

*T*he prime basis for reality revolves around each individual's perception of events in the surrounding environment. In order to understand a new substance, a scientist will subject it to every conceivable test: she or he asks, how does it withstand the elements? will it take an electrical charge? what are the constituents of its molecular structure? its organic structure? its emotions? how does its mind work? in what ways is it like me?

There is a certain similarity in the way a healer approaches a situation in order to understand an illness. Every avenue of human perception is probed by the inquiring healer, including the way of subjective, intuitive personal knowledge. Clues are sought for even the faintest hints of the underlying process: how does the ill person hold his body? what does the body itself look like? is there a structural fault, an indication of an imperfection, a weakening? does the way the body is held indicate a posture that protects sensitive or painful areas? what does the body itself feel like? the texture of the skin? the muscle tone? does the body feel vital?

An experienced healer will use every function of the five simple senses, but this is only the beginning of the search to learn how to alleviate the healee's condition. The need-to-help drives the quest to know, and so no avenues of awareness are left unexplored. Guided by a sense of urgency, out of the depths of the unconscious arise instincts that serve to unlock previously unused, or underused, doors to non-ordinary modes of perception.

With experience, one learns the value of extending the range of the common five senses as well as exercising latent senses. For instance, one learns to listen intently to nuances in the patient's descriptions of the illness and its many subjective effects. This sensitivity is called upon frequently, to acknowledge slight changes in the general level of one's own consciousness while in the act of listening itself. The body's potent private language, stimulated as interactions take place with the ill person, can be a fount of knowledge. This private language most readily translates itself through the functions of the autonomic nervous system. A cooling sensation alerts one that a fine wave of perspiration is taking the heat from the body, a momentary accelerated heartbeat warns one to be cautious, a sudden tightness in the solar plexus carries a message about potent emotions, a change in respiratory rate monitors the attention, etc. These cues, coupled with the sensitivities of various chakras, serve to effect a heightened awareness of self and other. Unless the healer learns to sort it out, she or he can be overwhelmed by the information load, which usually does not present itself so that it can be logically analyzed byte by byte.

The healing act itself programs its own conditions and style. At this time there is a way of knowing that is beyond mere information-gathering, an agile intelligence factor that leaps over the usual boundaries of structured logic and abruptly presents itself in a complete, total way. As quickly, the steps one has taken on this path elude the memory when one tries to consciously recollect just how this personal knowledge was acquired, how it presented itself so suddenly to conscious awareness. The very effort of capturing its processes seems, paradoxically, to assist in erasing the memory and retaining the mystery. During the process itself, one is momentarily aware of subtle cognitive senses coming into play. Somewhere in the multifaceted recesses of one's being there is a vaguely familiar, but impersonal, mind factor directing this deep knowing process. Full control is just beyond the grasp. Some of these impressions about the healee's condition can be objectively verbalized. As you hear your own voice relating these impressions and know them to be true, it is almost as if one is standing beside oneself. With something akin to awe, one hears as if from some source other than oneself, a well developed synthesis of information and an evaluation of the healee's condition.

Although it is happening to you—you are, in fact, talking about the ill person now, at this very moment—you yourself cannot believe it. There is a finesse to the skill of description, an elegant use of phrase that you do not usually associate with your modes of expression. Each time it is as though one were getting to know farther reaches of one's own consciousness for the first time. Each time, there are bits of the process that feel familiar. The total effect of this well organized, unified presentation of insights into the healee's condition can be truly awesome in its clarity and its fullness. It is as though you tapped a profound wellspring of singular knowledge about the individual that is all true. For instance, as the hand chakras move through the healee's field during Therapeutic Touch, one may pick up information concerning the onset of the disease process.

This access is not always "on." It seems most available to the healer during the healing act itself. Like the Muse, its special functioning seems to need special conditions and one wonders if it is the drive of the need-to-help that sets the tone for this evocation of personal knowledge.

FOSTERING LATENT SENSES

With the same insistence that calls one to give attention to the Muse, other attributes of the Self accompany the driving force of the need-to-help. These attributes are latent forms of personal knowing that the easy access of information in this high-tech age seem to make obsolete. Throughout history it has been known that these senses, called paranormal in our time, become more acute when attention is turned toward interior experiences, such as the healing act. At such times an active and conscious attention to inner cues can set up a standard for reality that becomes the criterion for one's personal life style. To pick up elusive clues to others' distress and to find within one's own consciousness the suggestions to alleviate it, the healer finds him- or herself honing the growing edge of these awarenesses that sharpen during these nonordinary states of consciousness. In the case where these communications with the inner self prove true, and the patient is actually helped by the knowledge, one is obviously likely to continue to evoke this personal means of information storage and retrieval.

It is the process of centering, which is at the core of such healing styles as Therapeutic Touch, that also serves to foster both the life-affirmative direction and the functioning of these extraordinary domains of consciousness. The ability to keep on center, to remain focused even under stress, becomes one of the hallmarks of the experienced Therapeutic Touch practitioner's way of life. Moreover, in Therapeutic Touch the initial assessment of the healee's energy state is made without necessarily making physical contact with the healee. As noted in Chapter 3, it is the nonphysical secondary chakras in the hands, and sometimes other chakras as well, that are highly functional during the healing act of Therapeutic Touch.

Chakras are centers of consciousness. As these centers are activated and their functions are integrated in a synchronous fashion, the harmonics of the shift serve to potentiate awareness of subtle phenomena. Latent facets of the human sensorium may come into being. Senses that rarely function in everyday life become actualized. Such activation further sensitizes one to non-ordinary states of consciousness: telepathy, by which one may come into mind-to-mind communication with other persons without regard to geographical separation; psychokinesis, the ability to move objects without physically touching them (considered by some theorists to be the basis of wound healing); clairvoyance and clairaudience, the ability to see and hear beyond the usual range of human perception; precognition, the knowing in the present of details about future events, and several other exotic states of consciousness.

The literature states that these non-ordinary states of consciousness arise quite naturally out of such practiced use of the chakras as occurs in the mature and conscious use of healing techniques such as Therapeutic Touch. As one gains mastery over these advanced states, they can be added to the therapeutic tools at one's command. Over the dozen or more years that I have been teaching Therapeutic Touch, I have noticed that some of these states occur quite quickly among those who regularly practice Therapeutic Touch. From written accounts in my students' journals, indications of the use of telepathy can be perceived on the average of two-and-a-half weeks from the time they put the healing techniques into consistent practice. Over time, experience with the healing act deepens. So does the conscious use of the chakras that give rise to these abilities. As noted earlier, this is one of the reasons that I have come to regard Therapeutic Touch as a yoga of healing.

RESEARCH CONTROL

One cannot intervene in another person's life, as one does when the charge is accepted to help or to heal, without convincing oneself that what is being done in the name of therapy is truly based on objective reality. Fantasy and wishful thinking have little place if valid healing is to occur. Nevertheless, one can succumb to their urgings quite easily and sometimes quite innocently. The control offered by contemporary research is considered by our society to be one way to assure a measure of validity and reliability to experience. One of the healing experiences that lends itself to a wide range of personal interpretation is healing at a distance, when the healer and the healee are geographically removed from one another. The healer is not at the scene where the healing action is taking place so the healer can create in his or her mind's eye any scenario. The situation, therefore, can be highly vulnerable to misinterpretation, illusion or even magical thinking. Traveling about a good deal as I do, I often attempt healing at a distance. From years of experience with meditations of several kinds, I have gained confidence in my own abilities. Nevertheless, the responsibility of teaching others what one knows stimulates a need for objective knowledge about the content. An opportunity to exert such research control offered itself to me in regard to one aspect of healing at a distance, the vivid visualizations that occur to the healer so engaged. It all started when I got to know, at a distance, a little mouse, Mouse #37.

AN EXPERIMENT IN HEALING
AT A DISTANCE

About ten years ago the Nutrition Institute of America under the directorship of Gary Null conducted the largest single experiment to that date on two modes of healing—healing by direct contact and healing at a distance. Mr. Null phoned me to find out if I would participate in the experiment. Since the study began during the rush of the final weeks of the winter semester, I confined my involvement to an aspect of the experiment that entailed healing at a distance.

By prior arrangement with Mr. Null, I received a photograph of Mouse #37, one of two mice assigned to me. The second mouse was not given a number, although it was stated to be Mouse #37's cagemate, and I assumed that it was a control. A brief letter of instructions asked me to keep a record of what I did. I was told that 174 genetically standardized mice had been injected with a highly virulent cancer virus and that the mice were not expected to live for more than three weeks. A total of fifty healers comprised the sample.

Since I ask my students to keep journals, it occurred to me to do the same. I drew up a list of what I thought might be useful data: date of each entry, the time, the context of the session, my daily activities, what I did (e.g., visualized), during the session, the content of the meditation that I did as part of the process, and other comments that seemed relevant. I continued to keep the journal for twenty-two days, although it was time-consuming. However, since I had no further communication from anyone connected with the experiment and feeling the press of other commitments, I finally gave up the journal, but kept up the healing at a distance for Mouse #37. My impression was that his cagemate had died several days into the experiment, but that Mouse #37 was well and hardy.

At the end of June I met a man at a cocktail party in San Francisco who was connected with the group doing the experiment. He told me that Mouse #37 was one of three mice still alive and that this mouse and one of the other two mice had no signs of cancer. I, of course, was delighted to get the news. I had been doing healing at a distance for my little friend and I continued to do so. In September—strangely, at another party in San Francisco (the study was being done in New York City)—I again received news about Mouse #37. He was well and very alive. Both of the other mice, however, had died. Later, a year from the initiation of the experiment, I heard from Mr. Null that Mouse #37 was still hale and hardy. This state continued for several months, until the following June. In response to a letter from one of Krieger's Krazies who planned to do biochemical studies of the effects of Therapeutic Touch, Mr. Null wrote: "Mouse #37 recently died of old age. It had lived longer than any of the other mice, and lived without discomfort and in a seemingly normal state of health."

The study gave me a great deal of satisfaction. In the year-and-a-half my interaction with Mouse #37 had become quite real to me and I learned a great deal from the experience. The really interesting part of that experience for me was the later verifications of several visualizations that I had noted in the journal. One visualization I had was a description of the laboratory in which Mouse #37 lived his days. I had occasion to go to the laboratory some months after Mouse #37 died, and Mr. Null took me on tour. The number of flights of stairs up to Mouse #37's room, the way the litter cages were stacked, the color of the paint on the walls, the spatial relationship of the door to the windows, and the direction of the building itself, all corresponded to my previously written impressions. Moreover, I seemed to have sensed several of the healers who were actually engaged in the study; that is, I had intimations of their presence in the laboratory in the early days of the study while I was in the process of doing healing at a distance. Later I was on programs with several of these healers in different parts of the country. These occasions gave me an opportunity to check out my impressions with them directly. The verification of visual impressions seemed to me to be the most significant aspect of my own involvement in this experiment. I determined to devise a research design that would test out these occurrences under controlled circumstances.

EXPERIMENT IN PERCEIVING AT A DISTANCE

I gave the name vivid visualizations to those mental representations I had perceived during the experiment with Mouse #37. On the basis of this experience I worked up a questionnaire to determine if such perceptions at a distance were prevalent among my professional colleagues.

Professional nursing care can be a highly personalized interaction between nurse and patient. When the situation is charged with feelings of deep concern about the patient as an individual, the caring nurse frequently discusses the circumstances relating to the patient's conditions with friends and family members during her or his non-working hours. The nurse may think about the patient in a concerned manner. Sometimes this concern is carried over the boundaries between the conscious and the unconscious mind and enters the nurse's dream life. It rises to consciousness while the nurse is doing routine tasks or in a frame of mind permissive to the perception of such imagery. To get a sense of the frequency of such occurrences I did an initial inquiry among 1,500 professional nurses in various parts of the country.

PILOT STUDY

In this pilot study about thirty percent of the sample (four hundred and sixty) reported that they had visualizations of their patients at a time when they were spatially distant from one another. Of this number eighty-two percent (three hundred and seventy-seven) stated that they also had the experience of unexpectedly perceiving a visual image, "within the mind's eye," of a sudden, crucial change in their patient's health status. Although they were unable to account for these perceptions in a conventional, rational manner, at a later date they found that the vivid visualization actually had occurred. Although there is considerable literature on the reception of knowledge, facts or data about events happening at a distance recently, these nurses had no acceptable way of communicating this information to their peers because there is no valid nursing theory that accounts for information transfers of this nature.

Visionary experience is ancient and is reported in all cultures of the world. In this country a unique feature of the Native American character is a strong dependence upon individual visions as basic guides in life decision. In Yoga, visualizations of persons or events at a distance are one of the *siddhis*, what we would call paranormal experiences, but which Patanjali describes as natural concomitants of the interior experiences of the yogi. Recent studies have indicated a significantly high correlation between compassion and a paranormal faculty called *psi*, an information-gathering process that occurs via no known sensory receptors.[75] It seemed plausible that healers working under the impetus of compassionate concern for people who were ill might have a high capacity for psi as vivid visualization.

VIVID VISUALIZATION

Visualization is a subjective process, and my memory of earlier psychophysiological studies on imagery and the visual process gave me the impression that there was a great deal known about it. However, a search of the literature revealed that although the ability to create a subjective visual reality is at the core of traditional Freudian psychoanalysis as well as more contemporary psychotherapies, its process continues to be inadequately understood. Just how we are able to create pictures in the mind's eye so that one thereafter recognizes a class of objects, whether those objects are objectively present or are an abstract symbol of those objects, eludes precise scientific explanation. This is a paradox, for scientific methodology itself relies upon visualization as an introspective act, i.e., the capacity to "see" a problem, the intuitive skill to clearly state a hypothesis, the capability to perceive an analysis of data, and the genius to "foresee" the inferences of research findings and so prepare a conceptual base for future studies.

A review of the current literature* indicates that it is limited; however, there are adequate indications that human subjects do respond in subtle but significant ways to information transmission over distance without the aid of technological devices. To date studies have not been done to determine whether the vivid visualization of information about events occurring at a distance can be used with reliability in a therapeutic milieu. The present report tests this hunch within an experimental-control design.[76]

The review of the literature made me cognizant of the work on "remote viewing" by Russell Targ and Harold E. Puthoff, physicists at the Stanford Research Institute,[77, 78] and also some of the controversy relative to material given to the judges that was provoked by that study.[79] In designing the study in Vivid Visualization I took care to learn from their experiences.

OBJECTIVES OF THE STUDY

In its final form the study had experimental and control groups of professional nurses and it was designed to test the reliability of their experiences in Vivid Visualization. At this time there was little other than anecdotal records to support or negate such extensions of consciousness as Vivid Visualization in a therapeutic milieu. Since such an experience among nurses, whether formally acknowledged

*A full review of the literature and the theoretical rationale of the study of Vivid Visualization will be found in Appendix F.

or not, may importantly influence nursing judgments about the nursing care of patients, this research was conceived as one mode of addressing the need for controlled studies of these types of phenomena. The specific goals of this study, therefore, were twofold:

1. To test the reliability of Vivid Visualizations that nurses have about hospitalized patients while these nurses were engaged in a meditative act at a place geographically removed from these patients, and

2. To evaluate this ability for Vivid Visualization against the ability of other nurses of similar experiential and educational backgrounds who would imagine the conditions, surroundings and interactions of comparable patients who were hospitalized in a remote location.

The more formal aspects of the research follow.

Definition of Terms

Nurse-Meditator: A professional nurse who has had previous experience with meditative practices of any kind. (See Appendix F.)

Nurse-Observer: A professional nurse who worked in a hospital and observed two in-house patients at stipulated times for three consecutive days in a specified manner. (See Appendix G.)

Patient: An adult or child hospitalized for any reason who gave permission to be observed for three consecutive days.

Meditation: The Nurse-Meditator:

- centers by non-forcefully quieting his/her thoughts and then thinking of the Patient by name.
- visualizes the Patient and then visualizes her/himself in the vicinity of that Patient.
- becomes sensitive to her/his own thoughts on how to be therapeutic to that person in the Patient's present condition.
- uses these cues as a basis for thinking therapeutically about that Patient. (See Appendix F.)
- records any occurrences of Vivid Visualizations. (For detailed instructions, see Appendix H.)

Vivid Visualizations: A spontaneous mental process in which a graphic pictorialization of an event arises to mind as if the visualizer is at the place of occurrence. Vivid Visualizations are recorded on detailed forms and are measured against the actual perceptions of the Nurse-Observer in additive fashion, according to the Hits, Misses and Items Not Perceived by the Nurse-Meditator, but seen by the Nurse-Observer. (Appendix H and I).

Imagining: A self-induced evocation of an image of a thing, a person or an event.

Hit: A correct statement about an occurrence at a distance.

Items Not Perceived: An event that occurs at the site of a Patient which is seen and recorded by a Nurse-Observer, but which is not noted by that Patient's Nurse-Meditator. The Nurse-Meditator is at a remote distance from the Patient during the occurrence of the event.

Miss: An incorrect statement about an occurrence at a distance.

Hypothesis

Hypothesis 1: There will be no difference between the means of frequencies of Hits, Misses and Items Not Perceived by Vivid Visualizations between three groups of professional nurses engaged in meditation of patients hospitalized at a distance.

Hypothesis 2: When these groups are combined into an overall Experimental Group, the means of the frequencies of the Hits of the Vivid Visualizations of the Experimental Groups will be greater than the means of the frequencies of Hits in the Control Group.

Hypothesis 3: The means of the frequencies of Misses in the Control Group will exceed those of the Experimental Group.

Hypothesis 4: There will be a significant difference between the means of Items Not Perceived in the Control Group.

Hypothesis 5: There will be consistency in the relationship of Hits, Misses and Items Not Perceived between the two Patients meditated upon by each Nurse-Meditator within the Experimental Group.

Statistical significance for testing the hypothesis was set at .05; that is, that there would be less than five times in one hundred occurrences that the result obtained by this study would happen by chance (see Appendix G).

Sample Characteristics

In its final form, the sample studied consisted of an Experimental Group of fifteen Nurse-Meditators and fifteen Nurse-Observers, all of whom were professional nurses who practiced Therapeutic Touch as an extension of their professional skills, and thirty hospitalized Patients. Initially these subjects had been evenly divided as three small matched groups. They all adhered to the same protocol, however, they were tested at different times, albeit under the same conditions. As will be noted below, under statistical analysis there was no significant differentiation between the groups and so their data was combined into one larger Experimental Group.

The Control Group consisted of fourteen professional nurses who had similar experiential and educational backgrounds to the nurses in the Experimental Group; however, none of them practiced Therapeutic Touch. Two of these nurses acted as Nurse-Observers on two hospitalized Patients. The remaining twelve nurses, at a site removed from the location of the Patients, imagined the conditions, surroundings and interactions of these Patients.

All nurses taking part in this study were graduate students at the Master's level (M.A.) who volunteered for this study. The participants were randomly chosen; all were women, except for one male nurse who was a Nurse-Observer in the Experimental Group.

All of the Patients had signed informed consent agreements; however, they were not told to which Group they had been randomly assigned. The Patients were all hospitalized at the time of the study, and the hospitals were all within metropolitan New York. The administrators of those hospitals were aware of the study and appropriate materials were presented for in-house research review boards as requested. There were no major delimitations to this study other than the requirement that the professional nurses who played the role of Nurse-Meditator have had some previous experience with any type of meditation.

Random Assignment

For each of the three small groups which finally composed the Experimental Group, random assignment to provide comparable numbers and characteristics in each group was done in the following manner:

1. Cards, each with the names of one Nurse-Meditator/Nurse-Observer pair, were put into a container,

2. The cards were drawn out of the container one at a time, and each pair was given a two-digit number beginning with 01 and proceeding in numerical sequence,

3. A Table of Random Numbers[80] was entered and the Table was read downwards, to assign pairs alternately to Groups,

4. Numbers were drawn until the appropriate amount of pairs for each Group was assigned.[81]

The Patients were within the normal workload of the Nurse-Observers in both the Experimental and the Control Groups. The Control Group of nurses were not selected in the same way as were those in the Experimental Group. In the Control Group it was the teacher who volunteered the classtime after obtaining the consent of the students in the class. The teacher was randomly selected from a group of such teacher volunteers. As noted above, these students' experiential and educational background was similar to that of the nurses in the Experimental Group.

Instruments

Since a study of this nature had never been done before in a therapeutic milieu, the investigator devised the instruments for the collection of data. Two forms were developed, for the Nurse-Meditator (Appendix H) and for the Nurse-Observer (Appendix I).

For the Nurse-Meditator, the specific data included information on any imagery, impressions, symbols or other visualizations that she experienced during each meditation. She recorded physical and emotional sensations that related either to herself or, in her estimation, to the Patient. Colors, sounds, odors and other sensory experiences were also noted. The Nurse-Meditator described her impressions of the physical environment of the Patient, i.e., the placement of the Patient's bed relative to the door and window, the kind of equipment that was in the room, etc. She drew a picture of the spatial arrangements of the Patient's room, if she could. The Nurse-Meditator was also asked to record her impressions of the Patient's physical and emotional states and his or her thoughts and interactions with others. Finally, the Nurse-Meditator wrote a judgment of how well she thought the experience went. Room was included on the form for miscellaneous relevant comments.

The form for the Nurse-Observer included questions on the demographic data of each Patient, the current medical diagnosis, the nursing assessment of the Patient's condition, a brief case history and summary of laboratory findings. The Nurse-Observer was asked to give a general description of the Patient's room and to draw a diagram of it. A description of persons who were significant to the Patient was also noted. The clock times at which he or she observed the Patient were recorded together with objective signs of the Patient's condition and behavior and any impressions the Nurse-Observer might have had about those factors. He or she also recorded any dreams or other subjective experiences that the Patient mentioned, and any activities and interactions the Patient had been involved in during the times of observation. Space was provided for the recording of other occurrences or impressions not covered by the study form.

Reliability and Validity of the Study

Validity of the contents of those two forms was provided by a panel of three professional nurses with Ph.D.'s who knew the authoritative literature. Construct validity was assured by having the forms used by both Groups. A measure of reliability can be inferred from the manner of statistical treatment of Hypotheses One and Five, discussed below.

Procedure

Initially three small experimental groups of equal size and equivalent characteristics engaged in this study under similar controls but at different times. Their data was later statistically tested for equivalence. The data of the three groups were combined and thereafter referred to as the Experimental Group. The Experimental Group consisted of fifteen teams. Each team was made up of one Nurse-Meditator, one Nurse-Observer and two Patients. Therefore, there were fifteen Nurse-Meditators, fifteen Nurse-Observers and thirty Patients in the Experimental Group. The Control Group consisted of two Nurse-Observers, two Patients and twelve professional nurses.

In the Experimental Group the Nurse-Meditator and the Nurse-Observer on each team did not know each other. The Patients were a normal part of the Nurse-Observer's work load, but they were not known to the Nurse-Meditator. The Nurse-Meditator and the Nurse-Observer communicated with each other only at the beginning of the study to decide upon a time that was mutually convenient, and for the Nurse-Observer to tell the Nurse-Meditator the names of the Patients and their medical diagnosis. Since the names of the Patients were known to the Nurse-Meditators, so too were their respective sex categories.

In the Control Group the two Nurse-Observers and the twelve nurses did not meet until the end of the study. The investigator told the twelve nurses the names of the two Patients and their medical diagnoses.

In each team of the Experimental Group the Nurse-Meditator did a meditation according to a protocol specifically set up for this study by the investigator (Appendix H).

This meditation was designed to simulate the concerned contemplation by the nurses of their patients, as was reported in the pilot study noted above. The meditation was done for each Patient at the time agreed upon by the team members on each of three consecutive days, and the forms were filled out after each meditation. The entire procedure took twenty to thirty minutes each day.

The Nurse-Observer unintrusively observed each of the Patients during the time of the meditation. Unknown to the Nurse-Meditator, however, the Nurse-Observer also observed the Patients for a minimum of five minutes in the hour preceding the meditation and also five minutes in the hour following the meditation. These additional times were included in the protocol to pick up possible incidences of time lag or time acceleration that might indicate precognition or postcognition in the Nurse-Meditators reports. The Nurse-Observer covertly took notes while in the presence of the Patient during the observation periods and filled in the forms in greater detail at a later time when not in the presence of the Patient.

No information was exchanged between the Nurse-Observer and the Nurse-Meditator or with the investigator until the end of the study. This was done so that there would be no unintentional exchange of cues. At the end of the study the Nurse-Observer and the Nurse-Meditator in each team met with the investigator. The data on the forms were then discussed in detail and this discussion was simultaneously tape-recorded.

In the Control Group the professional nurses were given the following instructions:

> I would like you to think about two patients who are presently hospitalized. Their names are _____ and _____, and their respective medical diagnoses are _____ and _____.
>
> Imagine what they look like, what it is that is happening to them at this time, their interactions with staff, relatives and friends. Imagine what their environments are like, their rooms, surroundings, equipment, etc. Note what they may be thinking about or dreaming of at this time and anything else that comes to your mind when you imagine these patients.
>
> Write as fully as you wish on the forms that have been given to you.

The forms were the same as those given to the Nurse-Meditators. While this was taking place, the two Nurse-Observers in the Control Group observed the two Patients in the same manner as did their counterparts in the Experimental Group. No time limit was given for the completion of the forms. When all were finished—a matter of about twenty-five minutes—the forms were collected and there was a brief recess. As investigator, I then discussed their experiences with the participants and this discussion was tape-recorded.

As noted above, in the Experimental Group the Nurse-Meditators and the Nurse-Observers followed time protocols that were different from each other to possibly pick up indicants of pre- or postcognition in the Nurse-Meditators' reports. There was a second difference between the Nurse-Meditators and the nurses in the Control Group. The former adjusted the time of meditation to the Nurse-Observers' schedule. The latter did their imaginings during their regular classtimes. Another difference arose unintentionally.

The Nurse-Meditators were meditating on patients who were actually ill. There arose a tacit, though never stated, assumption that the purpose of the study was to find out whether the Nurse-

Meditator's concentration of thought might in some manner help or heal the Patient. The investigator let the assumption stand, neither confirming nor denying it, until all the data were collected. This might be considered an ethical oversight. However, when the situation was weighed against the possible bias that further discussion of the assumption might have on the study data, I decided that the issue did not have a significantly substantive moral base.*

Results and Discussion

The data was analyzed in the following manner. For the Experimental Group, report forms of the Nurse-Meditator and the Nurse-Observer on each team were compared and rated for frequency of Hits (those items that actually occurred), Misses (those statements by the Nurse-Meditator that were not seen to have occurred), and Items Not Perceived (behavior of the Patient that was observed by the Nurse-Observer, but not perceived by the Nurse-Meditator). These data may be noted in Table 3.

For the Control Group the report forms of the nurses who imagined the Patients' conditions were compared with their Nurse-Observers' reports and were similarly rated for Hits, Misses and Items Not Perceived (Table 4).

The investigator's ratings were checked by a panel of experts and for this purpose the tape recordings of the discussions of the data between myself and the participants of the study, as noted above, were given to the panel for their review, as were all of the participants' original report forms. The level of statistical significance for testing the hypotheses had been set at p < .05. The rationale for this decision was based on the small sample size and the recognized complexity of predicting the behavior of even a small facet of human consciousness. However, as it turned out, the actual level of confidence for all of the hypotheses far exceeded p < .05. In fact, for Hypotheses Two, Three and Four the data demonstrated that p < .001, and Hypotheses One and Five were also strongly supported. The statistical analysis, therefore, indicates strong feasibility for further research on Vivid Visualization, using larger and more diversified samples and, of course, a more elegant research design that

---

*For a fuller presentation and analysis of the research data, see Appendix G.

TABLE 3

Raw Data of Nurse-Meditators in Experimental Group on
Measures of Hits, Misses, and Items Not Perceived on Each
of Two Patients

Nurse-Meditator	Hits		Misses		Not Perceived	
	Pt. 1	Pt. 2	Pt. 1	Pt. 2	Pt. 1	Pt. 2
1	15	12	5	3	4	3
2	9	10	0	0	1	3
3	6	8	2	0	2	4
4	12	10	1	2	2	1
5	3	3	1	2	5	3
6	13	9	0	0	3	4
7	5	7	1	2	1	4
8	8	8	3	1	1	2
9	8	4	0	0	2	2
10	6	4	0	0	1	2
11	3	8	2	1	0	4
12	10	2	0	1	2	0
13	10	4	0	3	1	2
14	5	3	0	0	3	1
15	9	12	1	2	4	2

would allow the multifactorial analyses that computers now do with ease.

A cursory glance at the raw data (Tables 3 and 4) may be of interest. It demonstrates a curious inverse relationship. While the Nurse-Meditators in the Experimental Group have a significantly greater number of Hits, the nurses in the Control Group have by far a larger number of Misses and Items Not Perceived. Discussion with these two sets of participants elicited a very different perception of what they were about. The Nurse-Meditators' Vivid Visualizations were unusually sensitive to the correct awareness of spontaneous and sometimes unexpected changes in their Patient's interactions and milieu. Visualizations based on the imaginings of the nurses in the Control Group stayed quite close to classical medical and nursing textbook descriptions of their Patients' medical diagnoses, which

TABLE 4

Raw Data of Professional Nurses in Control Group on
Measures of Hits, Misses, and Items Not Perceived on Each
of Two Patients

Nurse	Hits		Misses		Not Perceived	
	Pt. 1	Pt. 2	Pt. 1	Pt. 2	Pt. 1	Pt. 2
1	3	1	5	5	10	14
2	3	2	6	7	11	14
3	4	3	5	5	13	14
4	1	2	9	12	11	13
5	2	2	3	2	10	14
6	7	5	4	14	11	12
7	3	4	3	5	12	13
8	1	3	9	6	12	13
9	5	4	6	4	12	13
10	2	5	17	13	12	15
11	3	6	10	6	10	13
12	2	6	5	5	10	11

they had learned as student nurses. Contrary to these nurses' expectations, their Patients did not have these classical symptoms and behaviors to any significant degree. Therefore, their number of Misses and Items Not Perceived were up sharply from that of the Nurse-Meditators. It is possible that this strong reliance on textbook descriptions rigidly structured these nurses' imaginings. The conscious recognition of correct impressions they may have had were aborted when the impressions were other than what one would traditionally expect. To the contrary, the Vivid Visualizations perceived by the Nurse-Meditators, although they may not have been what they expected, were so *real* to them that they reported them as fact, and they were very frequently right.

All of the subjects in this study volunteered. However, the nurses in the Experimental Group volunteered by individual, unpressured choice, while those in the Control Group consented to take part in the study when asked to do so by an authoritative figure, their teacher. This might indicate a differential in motivation that needs to be explored further for its possible effect.

The Nurse-Meditators made out the report forms in the privacy of their homes; however, the nurses in the Control Group responded to the forms in their classroom. It is conceivable that they may have felt some inhibition in writing imaginative accounts in the presence of their professional colleagues.

The Nurse-Meditators had short periods of involvement in the study that was spread over three days, while the nurses in the Control Group responded during one extended period within one day. This overall longer exposure to the study of the Nurse-Mediators may have given them a better opportunity than their counterparts in the Control Group to feel comfortable with the stringencies of the research conditions.

In reviewing the data, the investigator recognized the possibility that the Nurse-Observers may have unintentionally acted the role of Transmitter to the Nurse-Meditators via a kind of mental telepathy. All of the participants in the Experimental Group were practitioners of Therapeutic Touch, which sensitizes one to experiences in interiority, as previously discussed. The Nurse-Observers knew the time of day or night that their teammates were meditating. They may have had strong motivations at those times for "their team" to be successful.

There was a strong sense of responsibility among the Nurse-Observers to be acutely aware of their Patients' relationships to environment and to others during the time of meditation. This sense of responsibility gave them a feeling of connection with their team Nurse-Meditators, so that at these times they reported a "felt presence" or "it seemed to me that she (the Nurse-Meditator) was looking through my eyes." Specifically, one Nurse-Observer stated, "I felt I was being used" by the Nurse-Meditator to perceive the Patients. All of these qualities—sensitivity to acts of interiority, being a supporter of the Sender (i.e., the Nurse-Meditator), the close identity with the Patients, and the recognition of being a link between the Nurse-Meditator and the Patients—are all acknowledged settings where telepathy may take place.

Finally, it is interesting to consider an unexpected feature of Vivid Visualizations. This is that transfer of objects of thought (or, as it is now dubbed, information), does not conform to laws of classical physics, which are concerned with the transfer of material objects. In fact, in this study there seems to be little relationship of a significant nature between the two. In general, the transfer of material objects over distance can be predicted on the basis of Newtonian mechanics; that is, a certain physical object placed in a certain situation will move in a certain way. This was thought to be true of everything in the physical world. However, the transfer over distance of non-material objects of thought—an image, for instance—seems to work more like the phenomenon of electric charge. The charged bodies (the Transmitter and the Receiver) do not need to be in physical contact in order to carry the charge (i.e., information), according to field theory. However, the literature notes that in experimental settings the information transfer process is not repelled by electric shielding. Therefore, one would not expect this kind of phenomenon to be fully explained by a model based solely on the electromagnetic field theory. Clearly the phenomenon is either the result of a field we have yet to define, or it is a conjunction of several fields, including the electromagnetic, that appear to accompany many human functions. It is left for further sophistication of research tools to clarify this issue.

IMPLICATIONS FOR PROFESSIONAL NURSING

The major implications of this research point to a need for the deeper study of acts of the unconscious among professional nurses. One of the predictable incidents in most nurses' lives is the trauma experienced as an immature student when one encounters the stark realities of life-or-death situations. It is the contention of many nurse educators that this initial shock importantly effects later learning experiences, has a profound effect on nurses' attitudes, and may in fact act covertly to influence the nurse to avoid such encounters in the future.

It is known that this exposure to traumatic human incidents is a crucial factor in the attrition rate of student nurses, and it may also be an important reason nurses leave the nursing profession. It is an inescapable fact that exposure to such stress significantly molds the personality and may affect the health of those nurses who are exposed to daily traumatic occurrences over prolonged periods. It is normal that our daily experiences may be repressed or simply forgotten. However, under emotion-laden circumstances, these repressions may become amalgamated with deep unconscious processes.

This study noted that Vivid Visualizations are a part of many nurses' experiences. The process by which this type of experience may occur is not fully understood at this time. However, authoritative literature indicates that it wells up from the unconscious. Further study of facets of the unconscious, such as Vivid Visualization, may help the nurse release repressed emotional content relative to his or her professional life, and elicit rich insights about human consciousness.

Information transfers of the kind present in Vivid Visualizations are frequently presented pictorally or symbolically, but not at the level of verbalization.[82] The recognition and further study of Vivid Visualization will help nurses to openly discuss their own and others' experiences. Acceptance of Vivid Visualization as a normal human potential will force the recognition of such possibility also occurring in their clients. This alteration of self-concept and concept-of-others may act to alter the basis of future nurse education, nurse practice, and research on both the nurse and on the nursing process itself.

I am convinced that Vivid Visualization is a natural human potential, as is Therapeutic Touch. This practice may be taught in the future in a controlled fashion with the development of appropriate biofeedback techniques. Physiological correlates associated with such information transfers are already known. From this study it seems that nurses who have a deep-felt concern for their clients, whether in their presence or at a distant site from them, would be prime candidates to bring this natural ability for Vivid Visualization into rapid actualization. However, it is also understood that nurses are not the only people who deeply care about others. Compassion is a generalized human potential. Therefore, all persons who actualize that potential for compassionate healing and concern also have a high potential for Vivid Visualization.

ADDITIONAL DESCRIPTIVE ASPECTS OF VIVID VISUALIZATION

Several qualitative aspects of this study appear to offer insight into the process of Vivid Visualization; therefore, it is useful to relate some of the study's descriptive materials. The clarity of the perceptions is quite striking. A report taken at random from a stack of papers at my side as I write turns out to exemplify this statement. The following reports of Nurse-Meditator M.T. were all correct. No attempt has been made to change the essential wording of the statements. M.T. has practiced Therapeutic Touch for several years.

Describing her method of doing Vivid Visualization, M.T. said, "I thought about the Patient by name, and immediately I was there, beside him." She visualized Patient C.B. as being a very young man with straight hair who was lying on his side. The sun was shining through the window, she correctly reported, and the bed was near the door. She perceived that a great deal of activity was going on in the room and that the doctors and nurses seemed to be working quite intensively on a patient in the other bed in the room. In actuality, this patient had just had cardiac surgery to establish a double by-pass in his coronary system. Several doctors and nurses were in attendance connecting equipment to the patient and getting him settled. M.T.'s assessment of C.B. was that he was a withdrawn person whose interests centered on himself. She visualized herself doing Therapeutic Touch to him. Her impression was that he seemed comfortable while she was working on him, but the pain returned later. The next day M.T. felt she had helped him get out of bed and sit in a chair. In actuality it was a small tub called a "sitz bath."

Although these were all high-quality Hits, M.T. herself did not feel that she was very good at Vivid Visualization. She was greatly surprised to discover her high degree of accuracy when her teammate reported her own observations. Synchronicity, one might think. However, as the following reports will demonstrate, the events are beyond mere random happenings. The Hits on M.T.'s second Patient were even more impressive. She correctly stated that the Patient, M.S., had a bed near the window and that she was lying with one leg slightly elevated on a pillow. M.T. felt that the Patient was very cheerful and kind, but that she kept people at a distance. M.T.'s impression was that "she (the Patient) needed to become accustomed to my presence." The Patient was very talkative, she noted, and liked to keep situations under her personal control. "She was a wary woman," M.T. said, "and cheerful only on the surface." The second day M.T. did Vivid Visualization, she perceived M.S. lying quietly in bed. She noted that the other bed in the room was empty. M.S. had been sleeping, she felt, but had been disturbed for some kind of treatment. It was reported by the Nurse-Observer that the doctor had changed M.S.'s dressing at that time. Nevertheless, the Patient was calm and thought her leg would improve.

The papers lying directly under M.T.'s report concern another Nurse-Meditator, D., who correctly described all of the following about a young male Patient, Patrick. D. visualized Patrick in a room with four beds, and his bed was on the right, next to the door. She said, "His problem is with a thoracic vertebra, and a brace holds his hand over his head." In actuality, his arm was in an overhead sling. D. felt that Patrick was talking to E. (the Nurse-Observer on her team) at a particular time, which was also correct.

G. and R., Nurse-Meditator and Nurse-Observer respectively, were a strange team during that study. G. was supervisor of an in-service teaching unit at the hospital where she was employed, and R., a male nurse, worked in the coronary care unit of a hospital many miles away. R. was the class skeptic and was quite reserved, cautious and pragmatic in his views. G., however, was in the throes of great change in both her lifestyle and her worldview, but she had not fully integrated these perspectives of life and living. She was still in the process of getting to know herself. They seemed to have little in common and did not know each other before the study. The day G. and R. reported on their experiences was the first time they had an extended conversation: "We had spoken fifteen words to each other in our whole lifetimes," said R.

G.'s Vivid Visualizations turned out to be remarkably accurate, although she said that while doing it, "I felt like a fool" and was threatened by the situation "because I didn't really know if my perceptions were right, and yet I had to go on." Her method of doing Vivid Visualization was "to attempt to put myself in the room with the client after centering myself. I used T.M. (Transcendental Meditation) procedures for five minutes. I felt relaxed and in a meditative state."

It is useful to look at her experience with one of her Patients in considerable depth. Because of a rapid turnover in the coronary care unit, R. had not been able to give G. the name of a Patient beforehand. The unit was so active he would have to choose the Patients on the day they would begin the study. Nevertheless, she correctly identified him as an elderly gentlemen, who was frail, had blue eyes, white hair, and a full beard. Although he appeared helpless in her visualization, he radiated a strong sense of calmness and serenity. He seemed very intelligent to her. She could not understand why she sensed that nobody talked to him. (He was a Jewish man and only spoke Yiddish, which nobody on that unit could understand.) She visualized that he was the only patient in a small room and was in a bed that was not near a window. There was a second bed in the room which G. said was empty. The patient had gone to the Recovery Room that morning. There was intravenous tubing inserted in his arm, but other equipment at his bedside was standard, not at all unusual. However, G. noted great changes in the bedside equipment the next day and correctly identified what they were. (The Patient had suffered severe pulmonary problems during the night and now had a tracheotomy with supportive ventilatory and suctioning equipment.)

G. and R. had agreed to participate in the study at 10 o'clock in the morning for the three days. However, on the third day G. had a prolonged staff conference and then forgot about the arrangement until she was on her way to lunch. When she remembered, her first reaction was casual; it was too bad to have missed the session, but nothing could be done about it now. However, it continued to dog her thoughts as she walked to the cafeteria. Finally, much to her own surprise, she left her companions and went back to her office to carry out the meditation, even though R. would not be there, she thought.

Strangely, in the meantime, at the hospital several miles away, the coronary care unit on which R. worked had become very busy that morning with an unusual load of emergency procedures. R. was under high stress because of the life-threatening nature of the problems. R.'s attention was caught up in the immediacy of the emergency situations which did not let up until lunchtime. On the way to the cafeteria R. realized that he had forgotten to do the observations that morning. However, the traumatic nature of the events he had experienced earlier were such that he dismissed the thought as being trivial. He found himself thinking, "Oh, the hell with it. The whole thing is silly. I'll just fake it."

Nevertheless, after a moment's reflection, he turned on his heel and went back to the unit to observe the Patients. In this way, although neither G. nor R. knew it at the time, R. was observing the Patients at the same time G. was doing the healing meditation. G. visualized a young man stopping at the doorway and talking to the elderly gentleman. She correctly stated that the young man had once occupied the other, now empty, bed in the room. He had been the older man's roommate. He had been transferred to another area of the hospital, and now was being discharged. He had stopped at the unit to say goodbye.) G. was perplexed because it seemed that the elderly man was possessed with the idea of obtaining a straw. As G. reported this, there was a highly audible gasp from R. It turned out that the doctor had told the Patient that he would remove the tracheotomy, if he could learn to drink with a straw. There were no straws on the unit at that time and R., returning to the unit just then, was recruited to go down to the Central Supply Room to get the Patient a supply of straws.

In her journal G. had written:

On Thursday evening I volunteered to be part of a project I did not fully understand. I said I knew how to meditate, but had I really been doing it? Not recently, that's for sure. In my notes I documented feeling ridiculous in my attempt to visualize clients I had never seen. I felt that my visualizations were all contrivances of a vivid imagination. Yet there was a strange feeling of peace and oneness with the clients and with the nurse, R., who cared for them.

When we reported on our experiences finally, there was nobody in that room more amazed than I at the results. I certainly did not feel that I had cured anyone, but I did feel a surge of confidence and validity that I had not identified with ever before. My faith in my own potential was not restored, I would say, but rather that at this late date it was truly initiated.

R.'s comment when he heard G.'s report was, "I am a little flabbergasted. Her descriptions are extremely accurate. How could that be?" In his journal he wrote:

G. and I had never spoken to each other before the Thursday evening in which we took ten minutes to agree on the schedule of observations. Apart from her knowing that I worked on a cardiac unit, she knew nothing about the patients I would be observing. At that time neither did I know this, since I had no idea which patients would still be on the unit the following Tuesday, the day selected to begin the series of observations. Our only other contact was when we gave our final report to Dr. Krieger.

I was utterly astounded at the accuracy of G.'s description of the Patients I had observed. I have never been skeptical of the assumptions that underlie the premises of this study. Rather, I felt that the real question touched on which of the experiences described in the reports could bear the weight of careful investigation and documentation. . . .

Sitting there listening to G. paint an almost perfect picture of the Patients, including their clothes, ages, personalities, lengths of stay and even snatches of things they said, placed me in the uncomfortable position of one who is at the heart of a profoundly moving experience, but wonders if those whom he will tell of it will believe what he is about to say. Boyd has captured my sentiments exactly:

> Had I been listening with all my intellectual analytic habits, this feeling would not have taken hold. I would have heard it too literally and gotten caught up in comparisons. But my mind was off-guard.[83]

Those last six words may be the key that will open my whole being to the "mysteries" present here. Truth, and those aspects of

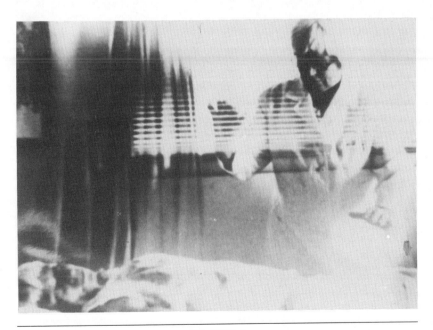

PLATE 4
Krieger taking her healing into her own hands—with
a little help from a photographer.

(Time-lapse photograph courtesy Betsy Ungvarsky, O.T.R.)

reality that we are not able to characterize, nevertheless undergo trauma when we listen too analytically, too intellectually—not because such reality cannot stand close scrutiny, but because our analytical faculties, our intellect itself cannot come to grips with the immensity of their being.

FURTHER USES OF THE VIVID VISUALIZATION EXPERIMENT

Because of the nature of this study, I have used it in one of my classes at the Master's level that focuses on healing as a professional therapeutic strategy. My purpose is to provide the students with an experience of research in progress by staging replications of the study with each new class. I never know how events will turn out, as every semester brings new students with unique complexes of variables. Nevertheless, each semester has produced unexpected reports on Vivid Visualization that support the original research findings.

To me, this attests not only to the reliability of the study, it forces the recognition of how little we understand about the capabilities of human consciousness. It is clear that the significant questions we each must face are: Are we willing to accept such power as a natural potential in humanity? Are we ready for the therapeutic use of the paranormal?

CHAPTER SIX

Therapeutic Touch as an Evolutionary Emergent

IMPORTANCE OF TOUCH IN EVOLUTION

*I*nvolved as I have been in the research, teaching and practice of healing, particularly Therapeutic Touch, for the past eighteen years, I have come to regard the posturing and functional use of hands in daily life with awe, admiration and curiosity. There seems to be a strong relationship between the fluid movements of the hands and the spontaneous expressions of the deeper levels of consciousness, so that these gestures constitute a descriptive body language of emotional attitude and mental set. I have always thought of the hands as being antennae for the brain, the expressive focus for the mind. As such I have come to think of them as the leading edge of evolution.

In the life sciences, embryology, the study of the development of the baby from conception to birth, has been considered to recapitulate the significant stages of human evolution. The growth and development of the child into the early stages of adulthood reflect the more recently evolved human functions. Embryologically, the exquisite sensitivity of the hand via touch derives from the ectoderm, one of the three basic germ layers of tissue of the embryo. Touch gives us more information than any of the other four major senses by allowing us to know in detail what is happening outside ourselves. Through touch we receive acknowledgment of other beings as physical realities. Touch allows disclosure of self, it allows access to non-verbal behaviors.

To the extent that embryological development does in fact recapitulate evolutionary development, one can see this evolution of touch reflected in the growing human fetus. In the embryo, the first of the central nervous system tracts to be myelinized (enclosed in a fatty sheath which serves to insulate the flowing nerve current, channel its energy, and make its conduction more efficient) is the spinothalamic nerve tract, which is concerned with the sensations of touch and pain.

While the fetus is in utero, the beginning of the primitive reflexes occur. Among the earliest is the hand-to-mouth sucking reflex, another kind of touch. At term, as the baby comes down the birth canal he or she is subjected to numerous subcutaneous stimuli. As the child is pushed against the sides of the birth canal it is touched repeatedly. Directly after birth, the baby exhibits the hand-mouth reflex which began to function while the baby is still in the womb. Over the next several week the child proceeds to other hand behaviors that help the baby explore its environment. This finally culminates in the hand-eye coordination which makes that environment the baby's own.

During the subsequent months of infanthood these primitive hand reflexes and their gradual release (so that the movements can be made voluntarily) underlie the psychophysiological development of the growing child. Although it has never been documented, it would seem that there are further hand behaviors that are age-characteristic up until at least young adulthood, for it is not until then that the process of myelinization is actually completed. One could also trace other characteristic hand behaviors through the latter part of life as various age-related disorders come into play. These include osteoarthritis, muscle weakness, slight parasthesias and tremors. Touch as a developmental phenomenon continues through the final stages of dying in a highly distinctive behavior. It is known so well that it has often been described in classical literature as plucking on the bedsheets. These little searching hand movements preceed the stillness of death.

TOUCH WITHOUT CONTACT

All of these hand movements are concerned with the tactile aspects of touch. What has caught my attention is that in Therapeutic Touch and similar other forms of healing, the healer may go beyond mere tactile functioning and use the hands in a wider repertoire of behaviors. Specifically, he or she uses the hand chakras, secondary chakras situated in the energy field overlying the palms of the hands, without necessarily making contact with the body of the healee. In this way the healer sensitively explores the overlying energy field of the healee for imbalances, blockages or dysrhythmias of energy flow. If the healer has mature abilities, he or she may also be sensitive to cues of a finer caliber of energy that seem to be concerned with the deeper psychosocial origins of the illness. To give a sense of the dynamic nature of this functional use of the hand chakras during my assessment of a healee in Therapeutic Touch, I shall describe in detail this process as I am doing Therapeutic Touch:

When I do Therapeutic Touch, even as I am approaching the healee I try to center myself, get in touch with all the "antennae" of my being, and fully sense how I can help that person. I also try to remember what brought me to this moment in the first place. I may even replay in my mind's eye the scenario that stimulated my first impulse to help or to heal. I remember the feel of that moment.

I align myself with the healee's energy level. To do this I center myself physically and emotionally. I consciously try to become acutely sensitive to subtle nuances in the energy flow between us, in the changes that I feel in that flow. These changes act as bits of information to me as I pick them up with my hand chakras. It is only then, when I am aware of this effortless alignment, that I begin to try to sense the problems of the healee.

I am now sensitive to any response in myself. These responses may be "gut" feelings, changes in cardiac rate, a tightness in the throat, or similar autonomic nervous system signs. I also sense any deviations from the feeling of dynamic alignment of the chakras themselves. This latter may make itself known in a feeling of actual movement—like a flip of the organic tissue—of the physiological solar plexus, or in a sense of fullness in the throat. This deviation from my own alignment may make itself known by an actual shift in consciousness whose occurrence cannot be attributed to the action of my own will. Accompanying this may come a keen perception or appreciation of the healee's problem.

The process of assessment does not proceed in a logical, straightforward manner, however. From time to time, as the imbalances and blockages in the energy field make themselves known, I try to deal with them to re-establish balance, rhythm and order in the energy field. As I work on the energy field I continually reassess those areas to determine whether my treatment of the situation has made a significant difference. It is at these times of reassessment that I will sometimes get a deeper sense of the problem or a cognition of other facets of the healee's field that may be in need of treatment.

This frequent reassessment seems to be important to me, for it is during these times that I get a sense of that person as an individual. I may pick up information about personal circumstances that occurred in the earlier life of the healee that were importantly related to the problem. It is also at this time that I may become aware of a strong personal linkage with that person on some level of consciousness. This sense persists even after the person and I are separated.

As I try to get a clearer sense of the dynamic within the person's energy field, I avert my gaze. I do not look directly at the healee. I look off into the distance, not actually seeing people or objects that may intervene in my line of vision. I use the screen of my mind as a background against which I try to apprehend, perceive, even, perhaps, to visualize the problem.

These realizations occur instantaneously, they are not thought through. They are often done in an atmosphere of some tension because the healee is ill or uncomfortable and I am trying my best to be helpful. The process seems somewhat analogous to what occurs when one wants to see some words that are all but illegibly written. One inclines the head and scrutinizes the paper, squinting with a concentrated gaze to get a better focus on the indecipherable information. So too, in the assessment I look into the distance as a mode of concentration and intently "listen" to the informing and envisioning apparatus, striving all the while to pick up these subtle energy signals. In the process I call on more than the usual five senses, however. For instance, although visualization is an important adjunct to the healing process, what is quietly transpiring between my hand chakras and the invisible web of the healee's field declares itself in other than visual ways. Here it seems that the consciousness of the chakras is the critical factor. Listening is a hearkening to clues couched in the faintest whisper in that silent communication.

Simultaneously, from time to time there is also a purely left-brained analysis, and an attempt to synthesize the incoming bits of data into a format that will make them understandable in terms of my previous experience and education.

Moreover, these experiences with the healee are not the same from day to day. Assessments at different times bring forth new information about the healee's changing conditions. As I have access to the deeper reaches of the field, I become more cognizant of the complexities of the healee's condition. I sense whether the data available have been correctly interpreted, and I feel a deep-seated, unmistakable inner acknowledgement of the clarity of the transmission of the data. On the other hand, there is also a clear indication (a wavering of decision, for instance) when I cannot understand all of the incoming data, or when the cues are beyond my ability to objectively comprehend their meaning. To be assured that I am working in the best interests of the healee, it is important to me that I honestly acknowledge these indicators. This objective attitude becomes particularly important as I continue to sensitize myself to this process of evaluation.

With practice, my insight may increase to the stage that I recognize quite different, novel, and unexpected ways of therapeutically treating the healee. The information that comes from the healee's energy field under these conditions presents itself with a surety that is, in retrospect, quite surprising. It is obviously important to judge the worth of these impressions in a most discriminating manner. It is here that an unbiased attitude free of personal prejudices is an ally of inestimable value. If I listen carefully to that ally, it tells me the truth.

EXPERIMENT WITH NON-CONTACT TOUCH

This ability to get information from the human energy field without touching the body of the healee, appears to me to have the essential characteristics of being an evolutionary emergent. It is at least one step beyond the striving for hand function that was the hallmark of previous human evolution. As such it fulfills a role as teleoreceptor, a receptor of stimuli at a distance, as are most of the other major senses of seeing, hearing and smell. In these teleoreceptors the object impacts upon the senses, although the object itself is at a distance. So, too, does the touch involved in Therapeutic Touch.

The idea that non-tactile touch may be an emerging, new form of human communication has intrigued me every time I have used it. Therefore, I developed a piece of research through which I could study this idea under controlled conditions.* In this inquiry I taught husbands, whose pregnant wives were learning the Lamaze method of prepared childbirth, to do Therapeutic Touch to their wives during the pregnancy. The premise of the study was that in doing Therapeutic Touch to his wife, the husband would significantly deepen his sensitivity to and awareness of both the mother and the growing fetus. As a consequence, a more caring, concerned, and satisfying relationship would develop within the family, I thought.

PILOT STUDY

A pilot study was undertaken on five married couples to test the feasibility of the proposed research. The wife in each couple was pregnant for the first time and was in the process of learning the Lamaze method of prepared childbirth. The husbands of the pregnant wives were taught Therapeutic Touch, which they practiced on their wives during the last trimester of pregnancy.

Summaries of individual interviews with each subject indicated that there was a strong general agreement among the wives that Therapeutic Touch is an intimate, highly personalized, sharing pair relationship that is very emotionally supportive and carries the connotation of caring. The summary of the interviews with the husbands stated that they felt that they had become more positive about the pregnancy and its responsibilities, more holistic in perspective, more concerned about the condition of their wives, and that there was a perceptible increase in their appreciation of both self and others within the family structure. This data indicated both significance and feasibility and a full-scale study was undertaken. The specific Therapeutic Touch techniques that were used in the study and the more formal aspects of the final research will be found in Appendices J–S. From a qualitative and humanistic perspective

---

*"Therapeutic Touch During Childbirth Preparation by the Lamaze Method and its Relation to Marital Satisfaction and State Anxiety of the Married Couple." The more technical aspects of this study will be found in Appendices J–S.

there were several changes in the husbands' attitudes that are of interest.

The first important change was, of course, the realization that, "you do not stop at your skin." As the husband began to explore his wife's energy field while doing Therapeutic Touch, he became increasingly aware of subtle differences in his wife's fields. Almost all husbands could learn to do this non-contact assessment during the course of one evening. In experiencing these other facets of his wife's being, he began to realize that this person he thought he knew so well had complex recesses to her personality of which he had not previously been aware. As he became more attuned and sensitive to her field dynamics he also became cognizant of a decided difference between his wife's field and that of his growing child. (The Lamaze method of childbirthing is most usually not taught until the mother is in her last trimester, which means that the fetus is between seven and nine months of gestation.) Finally, the father began to know his child in a very personal way during this period.

As he continued to do Therapeutic Touch during the pregnancy,

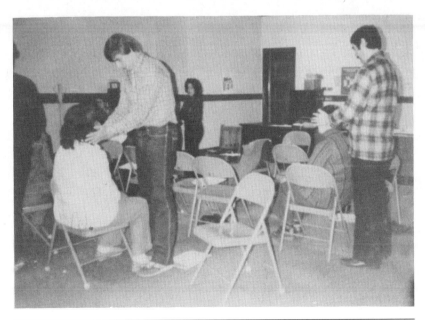

PLATE 5
Husbands giving Therapeutic Touch to their pregnant wives.

perceptions of the growing fetus' response to his touch deeply moved his emotions more directly than did the mere feeling of his child's kick against the inner wall of his wife's abdomen. The emotional impact of this first-hand experience with the gestating baby was frequently beyond words. However, one statement from a seemingly casual, macho husband captures the moment. "It's like that little baby just reached out and grabbed my heart," he said in unabashed astonishment.

Perhaps the most rewarding aspect of this study was that the recognition that you don't stop at your skin became a living reality. The way was open for the husband to come to the further realization that if there were no real boundaries or cut-off points to his energy field, it was also true for his wife and child. Frequently this acknowledgement led to an increased sensitivity to and understanding of each as an individual and as a family.

In the full-scale research built upon the lessons learned through the pilot study, the basic assumption was that this increased sensitivity would enhance family-centered psychodynamic relationships and reduce the level of the parents' anxiety. The research data supported only the former assumption, that the Therapeutic Touch practice would enhance the family centered psychodynamic relationships. The best predictors of this enhancement concerned the perception each had of the other's feelings and the ability to communicate with each other.

IMPLICATIONS FOR FUTURE GENERATIONS

The heightened sensitivity fostered by the Therapeutic Touch interaction lends indirect but substantive support to the contention that non-tactile touch can be regarded as an evolutionary emergent. It is a new wave of behavior in which a natural potential for increased human functioning can become actualized. This support is further strengthened by the ease with which many thousands of persons from many different cultures have been able to learn this manner of getting information that might otherwise remain imperceptible. The Therapeutic Touch interaction evokes strong emotional and powerful interactional response. The following excerpt from an article in *Glamour Magazine* provides an illustration:

It was incredible to me, says Abigail Mueller, twenty-nine. During my labor for the second baby, the nurse-midwife who attended me began Therapeutic Touch and the pain immediately changed to simple pressure. Her stroking over my uterus (without touching the skin), was much more effective than my Lamaze breathing. I just felt I could put myself totally in her hands and yield the discomfort to her.[84]

Acceptance of the therapeutic use of non-tactile touch is becoming common. People are just as ready for the emergence of novel human communicative functioning as they are to accept newly realized communicative interactions with dolphins and whales in the ocean and gorillas and wolves on the land. It is a matter of recognizing that the potential for change underlying the principles of human evolution is not worn out. There are potentials for the fulfillment of the human being that still lie dormant, like a story waiting to be told.

The emergence of the deeper reaches of self through the medium of helping or healing another is a choice for future human evolution. It comes from the most recent of generations. A good example is Carla, aged four, who is the daughter of one of my students and a second-generation Krieger's Krazy, indeed. Carla has observed her mother doing Therapeutic Touch since she was an infant. It came as no surprise for her mother to learn one day that Carla's peers had elected her resident healer of the nursery school she attended. It seems that Carla, emulating her mother, did Therapeutic Touch to all of the children who fell in the playground or otherwise hurt themselves. When asked what she wanted to do when she grew up, Carla had no doubt about her priorities. Without hesitation she clearly announced, "I want to be a healer, and a dancer, and a mommy." Who would want a better emerging spokesperson?

Carla is not alone, however. Stories abound. The following account serves to reinforce the argument for the increasing use of Therapeutic Touch.

A child of another of Krieger's Krazies is a few years older than Carla. She is at an age when children imitate their elders in earnest attempts to learn social roles. Her mother had heard that the children in the neighborhood had been playing doctor in a hut that had been built for them in a little grouping of trees. Torn between curiosity and concern, the mother decided to spy on the children.

Several times in the next week she watched the children unobserved. Each time she saw her daughter sitting against a tree a bit removed from her friends, who were indeed playing doctor. Her daughter seemed to be reading something that was totally engrossing. One day, cautiously approaching her daughter, she glanced over her shoulder to find her hunched over a copy of my book, *Therapeutic Touch: How to Use Your Hands to Help or to Heal*. She was deeply involved in practicing the exercises of the hand chakras!

She had been intrigued when her mother had done Therapeutic Touch, and, like Carla, she had wanted to learn how to be a healer. To her it seemed a most natural thing to do. There are untold learnings that uncountable ancestors have experienced over time that will support her natural acceptance of this most humane of human interactions.

I feel sure that she and Carla will be healers. I occasionally allow myself to fantasize about their future evolution, and that of their children. I consider the possibility of further psychological and cognitive evolution of children born into families that know for a fact that "we do not stop at our skin." They interact and build relationships accordingly. My wish is that they will freely allow this knowledge to shape, with great sensitivity for others as well as for themselves, the cultural mores by which they will live, as well as illuminate their conceptions about each other. Given these possibilities, the future seems worth the evolutionary striving.

CHAPTER SEVEN

Healing as a Lifestyle

FEW CONCLUSIONS, MANY QUESTIONS

I wondered what I could do that possibly might make a difference. I stood a bit to one side as a friend, Betsy, quickly moved down the hospital corridor toward a small female figure. She was indifferently clothed in the ambiguity of overly large, crumpled pajamas and faded bathrobe. Her problems, however, clearly declared themselves. I concluded that she had deep brain damage. My eyes swept over the contours of her body, uncomfortably twisted in a wheelchair. Both the upper and the lower extremities on her right side were tightly contracted in paralyzing spasm. Her head was constantly shaking in tremor, and the tone of her voice was flat, the words haltingly uttered, each sentence having a slightly rising inflection regardless of meaning. However, all that was quickly brushed aside as inconsequential in the exuberance and genuine affection of Betsy's greeting. We gathered up the supper tray and special utensils the patient had been using under the guidance of nurses watching from a nearby office, and wheeled her to the comparative privacy of her room. She and Betsy engaged in talk about hometown affairs, and I was content to sit quietly to one side and observe the interchange.

Seeing the patient up close served to reinforce my initial impression. I cringed at the images my memory conjured up of other brain-injured patients I had known. I thought of the predictable results of the neurological damage facing this young lady. An empathic surge lent urgency to my thoughts as I tried to sort out what I might do, where I might begin to be of help. I felt uncomfortable, inadequate and all but useless as I realized the odds against this person ever returning to the life of responsibility and independence she had known as mother, teacher, nurse, and social activist.

Suddenly my thoughts were interrupted when, as if from the depths of a long, narrow tunnel, a sentence echoed off the recesses of my brain. It was in response to Betsy's comment that she was looking better than when they had last met. The patient's words burst through my own thoughts, the closely grouped phrases resounding again and again within me. "But Betsy," she had said quietly, "How can it be that I am better when every time I look into the reflections in a cup of coffee, I see my head shaking? It didn't used to do that." I felt an aching wrench in the region of my heart as her words penetrated my consciousness and, without knowing how I got there, I found myself standing by her side, asking if I could try to help.

My hands moved rapidly down her sides, searching out an assessment of her condition. Her hand, I found, was contracted so tightly that her nails had bitten deeply into her palms. However, the Parkinsonian features of her neurological impairment made clear the need to start with the upper part of her field, in the area overlying her brain. I directed my attention there.

It is difficult to describe what I then did, and so a word of explanation is in order. Long ago I had realized that the mere three dimensions of length, breadth, and depth were inadequate to describe the inner experiences of the mind that accompany the healing act, that is, as I know it. In the living experience one goes considerably beyond the three physical demarcations of materiality to a mental act of interiority, which I have dubbed "going inth" to distinguish it from the dimensions of length, breadth or depth. I don't know—or care—whether it is a fourth, fifth or xth dimension-experience, but I do know when I get "there." Strangely, it is not difficult. One does not have to exert great effort to function therapeutically at this level of consciousness. What is demanded, however, is a clearly focused attention to the problem at hand once one is "inth." It is my impression that the more deeply I go "inth," the less effort I have to expend. However, I also find that the more difficult the problem is, the deeper "inth" I try to go. It is not a fantasy. It is a felt state of consciousness, much as is an act of deep concentration. Moreover, one sees its effects in the changed condition of the patient.

After working at that level for about ten minutes, in the intensive manner I described in Chapter 3, a shift in perception brought me to the realization that the patient's head was relaxed, quiet, and without tremor. I then turned my attention to her extremities. To my surprise, the disabled hand was no longer in spasm. I could gently and easily open the previously clenched hand. It stayed open and—biggest surprise—functional. The mask-like face now had expression, the skin was pink-tinged, and the eyes seemed to have luster. I taught her some exercises in imagery to reinforce the experience and her own empowerment. I spoke to her husband, who had come into the room in the meantime, and Betsy and I left shortly thereafter.

I had played it cool, I thought as I drove along the darkened parkway and Betsy and I discussed the experience from our separate perspectives. Nevertheless, for the next several weeks I continued to re-experience the interaction in my mind with a sense of immediacy and satisfaction that I could not deny. However, neither could I deny that the analytic side of my nature continued a barrage of questions about the apparent healing. The insistent inquiry was a constant companion whenever my thoughts recollected the incident. It was not that I doubted what had occurred; after all, there had been witnesses. However, unless I knew for sure that the improvement in the patient's condition had lasted, then what I had done was not really very much. What puzzled me, and continues to puzzle me, is the nature of the healing act itself, the truly effortless effort that is its hallmark. It is invariably available to help, if not to heal. It is rarely tiring, and it is a most rewarding personal growth experience into extensions of the deeper consciousness. But why was it so easy? queried my left brain.

The experience had been deeply gratifying and as I thought about it, I felt a glow; nevertheless, when I reflected more fully upon the incident, I also was aware of unease. I thought it was because a calendar full of prior commitments did not allow me the time to return to the hospital for further interactions and closure with the patient. When I finally had time to sort out the experience more thoroughly, however, I became consciously aware of the effect the strong emotional content of the occassion had on me. I realized that it had acted as catalyst, giving form to a clutter of questions that had clamored for my attention over time. The questions had nothing to do with my sense of validity of the experience but, rather, the thoughts were tinged with the excitement of the chase of a new idea or of a widening perspective of the possibilities of healing. It is the thrill of pursuit of the unknown that can become the hallmark of the researcher who enjoys matching wits against the strongly specified question, rather than being content with a relatively generalized answer. The very act of trying to systematize the questions lent coherence to my wonderings and structure to my quest for meaning.

The basic problem in understanding the healing act is that the prime actor, the healer, does not understand in detail what it is he or she is doing any more than a youngster knows the particulars underlying the success of riding a bicycle for the first time. The answers to both cases in response to the question, "How does it work?" would be: by the seat of the pants. The ready answer by those who purport to know, is in terms of healing energy. However, the pragmatist wants to know what kind of energy *that* is, and that is difficult to specify. Perhaps the difficulty lies in the nature and the paucity of our knowledge. This knowledge is limited by the strictures of our conventions on how questions may be stated, and what can be questioned.

It is the ability to repattern human energy that seems to be at the basis of the healing act. Energy is a gross term, however. In classical physics energy is considered to be the movement of molecules. In solids, these molecules are deformed by the gravitational field. In liquids they flow in response to hydraulic pressure gradients. Gases are thought to be able to travel indefinitely, if unconfined. The radiations of light have a motive power per second that serves to delimit the workings of the universe, as we presently understand it. These characteristics of the movement of molecules within the known media can be measured and, therefore, constitute the accepted context of what energy is.

Within this frame of reference, the term "healing energy" has little meaning. Although, I would think that if a wound is healing, tissue is regenerating and therefore certainly "work"—the criterion for measurement in the physical sciences—is going on. There are, nevertheless, valid confounding variables that serve to considerably complicate matters. In the early research I did on blood components of persons treated by the laying-on of hands and, later, Therapeutic Touch, one of these intervening variables is time (the effect of our relation with circadian rhythms), another is timing (the effect of synchronization of the "ten thousand and one" factors with which we interact daily).

There are many other complex but subtle factors that are part of the healing process, yet difficult to assess. For instance, at this time psychosomatic problems constitute the greatest proportion of illness in the world. Depending on who you read, it is estimated that between 50% and 80% of all illnesses in the world are considered to be psychosomatic in origin. There are very few "bugs" left today. Most illnesses, even in Third World countries, are caused by stress. Therefore, stress-related illnesses are pandemic. The array of physiological dysfunctions that are related to stress can be shocking, until one stops to consider the innumerable physical and psychological pollutants that press our planet and its people to the limit every day.

Studies have shown that stress significantly alters blood supply and blood pressure, respiratory rate and pattern, digestive processes, and neurological activity. And—most important—stress interferes with the immunological balance of the body itself.[85] Two of the systems in the body that are central to the maintenance of immunological balance are the autonomic nervous system and the endocrine system. Both of these systems have been shown to be chemically sensitive to the healing process in Therapeutic Touch, acupuncture, biofeedback, and imagery. However, there is no acceptable theory of just how that occurs. It is as difficult to know *why* healing occurs as *how* healing occurs.

THE POSSIBILITY OF PLACEBO THERAPY

The vehicle most often pronounced responsible for the healing process is the derogatory term, the placebo effect. The placebo effect is believed to be based on suggestion. In the classical case of placebo therapy, an ill person is given a pill or an injection to ease a medical problem. The substance is in fact inert, very frequently being no more than harmless salt water, or a sugar pill or powder. It is given by a powerful or influential figure who suggests to the patient that it is an effective drug or medication for the ailment. That figure acts as a placebo. The belief in the efficacy of the placebo often enables the patient to mobilize his own innate abilities to counter the symptoms by altering the actual biochemical and psychosomatic responses of the body. This has been verified, but little understood.

Murphy lists some of the known effects of the placebo response. Placebo has been known to significantly assist in the reduction of both fat and protein in the blood, change white blood cell levels, reduce the trembling associated with Parkinson's disease, relieve depression, increase sleepiness, lower the subjective level of post-operative wound pain, lessen the painful symptoms of arthritis, "eliminate the symptoms of withdrawal from morphine and produce various specific effects [found in] both stimulant and depressive drugs."[86] In reviewing the list it is difficult to discern a specific underlying physiological or psychological system which might be the common denominator of this very broad spectrum effect.

Studies that have pitted tested pharmaceuticals against the placebo have demonstrated the overriding power of the placebo effect. Wheatley's famous study on the use in general medical practice of psychotropic drugs is but one example among a growing body of evidence.[87] Wheatley found a 50% therapeutic response—which is at least as good as random expectations would offer—in patients given placebo. This compared to a 75% response—which, in this sample, was barely more significant than chance expectations—in patients given known psychotropic drugs. Since chance expectations are what one would expect to happen, regardless of what the drug was, the inference is that there is little difference between the effect of psychotropic drugs, which are medically dispensed by the millions every day, and a placebo.

The placebo effect has been recognized to be potently related to the biochemical production of endorphins in the brain, by which the experience of pain is dulled. Considered from this perspective, the placebo effect is now gaining recognition as a powerful way to mobilize the individual's capacity for self-healing. However, this was far from the thoughts of those who first introduced the idea of placebo.

MISTAKEN ATTITUDES TOWARDS PLACEBO

The medical use of autosuggestion was first reported more than fifty years ago by Evans and Hoyle in reference to its effects on patients with a particular cardiac problem, angina pectoris.[88] The term "placebo effect" was given to its use. The recognition of its

apparent importance led to its central placement in the pharmacological model for testing drugs in double-blind studies. Double-
blind studies are designed to eliminate the possibility of suggestion
by assuring that neither the patient nor the experimenter knows
which pills contain the medication that is to be tested, and which
is placebo. To further tighten the research design, patients were
used as their own controls. This was also done in the study depicted
in Table 2. This was a hematological study done on patients treated
by the laying-on of hands and by Therapeutic Touch. However,
about twenty years ago confidence in this cross-over design was
undermined by observations and reports that both the medical and
nursing staffs were strongly influenced by inference and suggestion
during these tests. Even more unexpected have been reports in the
past decade of significantly higher than chance findings of statistical
errors and research flaws in studies published in the foremost medical journals in both the United States and Great Britain.[89] These
findings have not had wide circulation, although they are valid. The
pharmacological model (the placebo effect) is still perpetuated in
clinical research and the term "placebo" continues to have a dis-
paraging connotation.

Both placebo and autosuggestion can act to stimulate self-healing,
even if the details of that healing process are not understood at this
time. I was appalled a few years ago to see for myself the senseless
defamatory effects the continuance of this model can have on in-
nocent persons.

Shortly before I was scheduled to leave for a lecture and workshop
series abroad, I received a request from a psychiatrist to consult
with her on one of her patients, a nurse, while I would be visiting
her country. My schedule was such that the only time I could meet
with her and her patient was during a workshop lunch break. The
patient had been highly regarded in her profession when she returned from a vacation in Mexico two years before our meeting.
Since then, she had been plagued by lethargy, generalized pains,
and a sense of exhaustion following even minimal effort.

The hospital administration at her workplace became increasingly
concerned as physician after physician—six in all—could find nothing clinically wrong. After subjecting her to several tests, which
were all inconclusive, they referred her to the psychiatrist as a placebo maneuver. The psychiatrist had been working with the young
woman for several months. At this time her conclusion was that

the patient was psychologically sound. She herself did not know how to help the patient, who still had the symptoms.

I approached the young nurse and talked casually with her and the psychiatrist, explaining what I would be doing in the assessment. The patient was in her late twenties, and seemed intelligent and attractive, except for her eyes, which lacked luster. The orbits were darkly rimmed. I had expected complex problems, in view of her history. Therefore I was startled when I immediately found a significant disturbance in the area of her energy field overlying her throat chakra. I then brought my hands into contact with her neck and physically palpated the tissues. Surrounding the thyroid gland was a large, hard, immovable mass that penetrated into the surrounding tissues. My own hand chakras register in a distinctive manner when tissue I assess through Therapeutic Touch has malignant growth. With some concern I reassessed the area and then her whole energy field to thoroughly check my findings. When I felt quite sure that the growth was malignant, on some pretext I took the psychiatrist aside and told her of my findings. It happened that there were eight physicians attending that particular workshop. I asked that we not tell the patient until I had time to ask several of the physicians to check my findings by physical examination. In a short time the workshop participants returned from lunch. I asked several of the physicians to examine the patient. To my dismay, they concurred with my assessment. The psychiatrist and I then spoke to the patient privately.

We started cautiously by underlining the tentative nature of my findings. They had not yet been corroborated by laboratory reports. Tears came to the young woman's eyes and I readied myself for crisis-interventive techniques. The crisis was of a nature I had not anticipated. Clasping her arms tightly around her own torso, she exclaimed, "Thank God, it *is* physical! It's an actual, physical problem! I have been driven almost mad by the constant insinuations about my character and my emotional stability these two years. I can face the challenge of cancer, but I can't continue to face the aspersions that have been directed at me so callously."

The psychiatrist and I had difficulty looking each other in the eye out of shame for our peers in the health profession. It was incredible that a mass that was so obvious should have gone unnoticed for so long. It was unconscionable that reliance on medical technology had not been humanized by the physical touch that could have found the problem so easily. It was frightening that a psychiatric diagnosis was made so insensitively. Looking at the young woman who had been hounded by the undeviating, searing accusations of authorative figures, I realized that this was an utterly pitiful situation built upon ignorance and indifference. It had no place in a professional field intended to meet the health needs of the people.

PLACEBO AS SELF-HEALING

One wonders why it has taken so long for society to perceive the inferences of the placebo effect in a constructive way, for the placebo indicates the large potential we each have for self-healing. The literature on the use of placebo in research demonstrates a potent human-to-human sensitivity. Numerous studies have revealed the strong influence of suggestion and inference on mind-set. More remarkable are the studies that indicate the significant effects one's thoughts can have on another person. Even more astonishing are the lengthy lists of physiological and psychological functions attributed to the placebo effect, as noted above. Placebo effect is no less than the ability to generate within oneself a repertoire of factors that contribute importantly to self-healing. The powerful effect of imagery on the immunological system has now been supported by valid research. Why shouldn't other aspects of autosuggestion be acknowledged for the therapeutically potent effects they can have, particularly in psychosomatic illnesses? Properly directed, one could learn to use these forces for life-affirmative purposes.

EMPOWERING THE PATIENT

Information about these possibilities should be shared with those in need, the patients. They could then ready themselves for important personal growth experiences. When I was making my rounds as a supervisor of nurses in a hospital, I would often reflect on the heroic courage of many of the patients. Had they known the inner way to intervene in their own illness, they would not have waited for medical permission. They would have made the most of the secrets from the labyrinths of their own minds. What a triumph that would have been for them! Why didn't we encourage and facilitate their own powers of self healing?

We do not strongly empower our patients in the interests of their own well-being. The more thoroughly and consciously healing becomes part of one's lifestyle, the more clearly it is perceived that in the last analysis it is the patient who heals him- or herself. Once this is accepted, the healer's objectives also become clarified. These objectives are threefold. The first is to bolster the healee's own potential for self-protection through the strengthening of that individual's immunological defenses. The second is to support the natural intelligence of the body towards self-healing. If those lines of defense are adequately supported and there is a therapeutic response, then the third objective is to educate the healee in preventive techniques that will serve in the maintenance of a state of high-caliber, vibrant well-being. The healer can create a therapeutic milieu that encourages the healee towards a direct, personal relation with the internal workings of his or her own being. If this can be done in a manner that awakens the individual to an awareness of personal, intrinsic wholeness, I would call that a good day's work.

ORDERING PRINCIPLES OF THE HEALING ACT

At the crux of maintaining a healing stance in one's lifestyle is an acceptance of ordering principles that may be perceived at work during the healing act. These ordering principles can also permeate one's own day-to-day actions and give them a context in which the meanings of those actions become apparent. There is elegance, beauty and an indescribable grace in the harmonious regularity and appropriate specificity of the healing process in action. This process is truly awesome to witness. Watching it work its unique magic, one wonders over and over again: how can healing be so selective as to inhibit the chaotic growth of tissues in malignancies, and yet vigorously stimulate the precisely ordered laying-down of new tissues in wound healing? What is the nature of this healing energy that escapes the definitions of science? The healer has cause to wonder, as well as the scientist. It takes a special kind of courage and/or sense of commitment to allow such a powerful unknown to become the basis of life decisions.

When one's life has such a focus, everything else acts in relation to it. Mandalas (patterned wheels or circles of concepts or symbols) are used in many cultures as visual aids to focus the attention during acts of contemplation. When patterns of the ordering principles that underlie healing become apparent to the person intent upon the healing way, these patterns of thought and behavior are used as the hub of the wheel. They form a central point around which one's quest for meaning gains structure, and the contemplation of that meaning gains depth. When awakened, in one of those mysterious acts of the human psyche, this interior structuring of itself may act as a focus for self-healing. The center becomes a point of reference for the consciousness, and so becomes itself a source of energy available to the individual. Within its sphere of influence, relativity is its theme. One seeks meaning out of the diverse, seemingly random events of life. In the functional use of the ordering principles of healing as the context for one's lifestyle, one begins to perceive possibilities for valid integration of apparently inconsistent, irreconcilable, or incongruous factors as their patterns are fitted together in relation to one another. In lockstep with this relativistic mode of working out meaningful solutions to conflicts, one's perception of reality undergoes conversion. The focus comes into resolution amid the many daily life activities. The unmistakable marks of these universal principles of order make themselves apparent.

Healing, in which one is deeply concerned about the well-being of another, facilitates this shift in perception. Under the promptings of compassion, there is a relatively effortless transition from the limited, egocentric internalization common in our competitive society, to a more open, humanistic reference to the self. A concern for other is a concern for self. Thus, healing as a lifestyle is urged on by a driving quest for meaning. Meaning, as reflected in the ordering principles that underlie the healing process, is clearly spelled out under the precise tutelege of a persistent reality whose center is everywhere and, therefore, is everywhere accessible. This is, of course, but one person's interpretation of life experiences, and as such it is no more than my opinion. As opinion, the hope is that it will be "held in the hand, but lightly"; that it will be grasped in such manner that it can be relinquished, if need be, when other points of view appeal to one's intelligent consideration.

"Listening" to Oneself: A Tool for Self-Awareness

INTRODUCTION

*T*hree characteristics of the person who does Therapeutic Touch successfully are:

- intentionality
- motivation in the interests of the healee
- an ability and willingness to confront oneself with the question: Why do I want to be a healer?

It is frequently difficult to evaluate ourselves in these areas, for all three characteristics are deeply embedded in the unconscious, which is little understood in our culture. The following self-awareness techniques are suggested to help you uncover this information so that you may fairly judge yourself in these areas.

Note: Accept the material as a true evaluation of your thoughts and feelings about helping people. There is no need to make decisions about what to do about your attitude toward helping people unless you want to do so. The purpose of this tool is to help you clarify the issues and to acknowledge them.

INSTRUCTIONS

Carry a small pad with you for the next week and note in it the following items whenever you think about helping somebody:

1. Be aware of the feeling tones of your body. Ask yourself: Am I feeling sympathetic to this person's condition, or angry that it has to be me that is helping him or her, or frightened at the responsibility it may entail?

2. Be aware of what your body is telling you about your thoughts of helping another. Be aware of your body posture and ask yourself: Do I feel any unusual pull on my muscles or tension within my body? Do I feel any unpleasant sensations? Of what pleasant sensations am I aware?

3. Be aware of any memories that arise when you think of helping someone. Do you have fantasies at this time? Do you talk to yourself about it when you reminisce or fantasize?

4. Allow yourself to fully experience your physical and emotional reactions. Identify the ideas and feelings that arise and then write them down.

Do not reread your material immediately. Wait a few hours or until the next day to review what you have written. At that time analyze the information that you have found about yourself. It may help you analyze the material to speak the words you have written into a tape recorder and then replay it.

Visualization of the Dance of Energy Forms

E nergy is ubiquitous. As Einstein discovered, $E = mc^2$; it is every-where and everything. It looks various: like a fiery incandescent flash set free against the open sky, like black smoke boiling out of man-made smokestacks, like a piece of iron rusting unnoticed by the wayside. It is not physical only; it runs the gamut of emotions, of thoughts, of imagination, and perhaps of aspiration. It is the stuff by which we live and by which we die, the basis of all experience.

Energy is so ever-present that we become indifferent to its many guises. At the split second of critical mass, in a nanosecond, or in a wink, it can change into a thousand-and-one things and then change again and again. Below are words for different kinds of energy manifestation as they are caught in the rigid mesh of time and space (an illusion, of course). Look at these words as if for the first time. Give free rein to your imagination, and be sensitive to the visualizations that spontaneously arise as you consider these names one by one. Jot down on paper, or speak into a tape recorder, or sketch, or write a haiku, couplet, or short poem about your

Note: It is this dance that is at the heart of human growth and development. T.S. Eliot wrote of the cycles of life, "And all there is is the dance." Do you agree?

impressions as you glance at this list and as the many forms of energy dance before your mind's eye:

rays	pulsations	sprays
streaks	groundswells	swirls
bursts	wavelets within waves	rushes
thrusts	ripple effects	floods
projections	thrills	ebbs
outpourings	shimmerings	flows
	iridescences	tides
		currents

APPENDIX C

Exploration of Personal Field Dynamics

*F*or an understanding of the basis of this exercise, see Chapter 3, "A Yoga of Healing." The underlying assumption is that emotions are the patterned flows of energies within the psycho-dynamic field. The task is to bring attention to these patternings, to allow them to well up to a conscious level, and perhaps thereby to provide insight into our own feelings and thoughts.

1. Sit in a comfortable position and center yourself; that is, gently come into contact with an inner sense of yourself. Pay no attention to noises or movements in your environment. Do not force your attention; acknowledge that there are noises but that for the next few moments you want to fully appreciate your inner quietude. You may find that you do this best with the eyes closed.

2. From that center, move within your body as a consciousness, getting a personal sense of self without restriction, without tension. However, retain the integrity of yourself as an individual.

3. Now turn your attention just outside your physical form and get a sense of your consciousness that just beyond your skin.

4. Breathe in a natural, comfortable manner. At a moment that seems best to you, on exhalation, suffuse this area just beyond your skin with an energy mode of your choice—light, color, song or breath.

- If your choice is light, experience it as a transparent luminescence.

- If your choice is color, experience it as clear, vivid, and radiant,
- If your choice is song, fully experience its vibration and the lilt of its rhythm,
- If your choice is breath, upon exhalation experience it as as a surge of life-enhancing energies.

Whichever energy mode you choose, keep the energy moving toward the periphery, away from your physical body.

5. Keep sensitive to the energy flow, and note any variation in that flow.

6. Also, carefully note any impressions you have of words, images, colors, sound, and the like as you gently go out—feel your way—into the farthest reaches of your psychodynamic field.

7. When you have gone out as far as you can, explore your field. Write, using words or symbols, or draw your impressions as fully as you are able to.

8. Rate your impressions on a scale from 1 to 5 according to how meaningful the impressions are to you, with 5 as the most meaningful.

9. Note also any physiological and/or psychological reactions as you set up your rating scale, and record a description of them.

10. Take the writings or drawings that you gave a rating of 3 or more and, using free-flow or stream-of-consciousness writing, compose a short essay or poem on their relationship to each other. Put down everything as it comes to mind, even if it does not make sense at the time.

11. Put the material away for two or three days. Then, at a time when you can be by yourself for a short period, read all the material you have written or drawn. In the margin of the paper note any association of ideas or any other relationships that come to mind. Analyze the content of your impressions and write a short paragraph or two on any insights that occur to you.

12. Act on those insights. Their validity will present itself to you in your life.

APPENDIX D

Exploration of Others' Field Dynamics

For an understanding of the basis of this exercise, see Chapter 3, "A Yoga of Healing." The underlying assumptions of this exercise are:

- Man is an open energy system.
- Emotions are distinctive, patterned energy flows in that system.
- These distinctive patterns can be distinguished by empathic persons.

1. Choose a partner and decide which of you will be Transmitter and which will be Receiver.

2. The Transmitter should sit comfortably in a chair, and the Receiver should stand behind the Transmitter.

3. Both should take a moment to center. Then the Receiver should place his or her dominant hand about two to three inches above the Transmitter's shoulder with the palm of the hand down.

4. The Transmitter should remain on center, accepting of the Receiver. The Receiver also remains on center and open or neutral to the Transmitter.

5. From the moment the Receiver places his or her palm in the Transmitter's field he or she should be sensitive to any cues that come to mind—words, symbols, pictures, colors, sounds, mood, emotion, and the like.

6. After about two minutes the Receiver should write down as fully as possible whatever cues were picked up.

7. The Receiver and the Transmitter should change roles.

8. When both have finished, they should discuss their impressions with each other.

9. Score one point for each Hit (correct impression); score zero for each Miss (incorrect impression).

Below are letters from students who have tried the above exercise.

Dear Dr. Krieger,

I recently attended your workshop on The Therapeutic Use of Paranormal Phenomena. In the workshop we did a exercise of putting our hand on our partner's shoulder and verbalizing our images. At the time my partner could not relate to what I had visualized. I received a letter from her a few days later. I thought that you might be interested.

Sincerely,

Patricia

Dear Pat,

I just had to write! Remember the exercise we did where you picked up the images of duck, bird, horse, clown and bright colors, and lots of activity? Well, after spending some time with my friend that evening (I checked out all her paintings with no results) I got home at about 11 P.M.

Right in our living room (which really is *now* the children's playroom) was the whole scene. John and the kids had had a wonderful afternoon rearranging some of their toys. They had put them all up on our two side windows. . . . There they were: the duck and the bird; and the clown marionette (which usually is upstairs) was hanging down from the bamboo shade. John had planned to bring down the hobby horse from the attic, too, but things got too hectic.

He said they all had a great time deciding how to place the toys on the windows and sills. I asked him what time they had gotten involved in all the decorating, and he said about 2 or 3 P.M. About the same time we were practicing the exercise!

I don't know how it all fits in or if it was just coincidental, but I was a little flipped out over the whole scene. I kept saying, "Here it is, the duck and the clown." John kept saying, "What are you talking about?"

You were quite perceptive, if it all has any relatedness. Anyway, I thought you'd be interested to hear!!

Danielle

APPENDIX E

Human Field Holomovement

*F*or an understanding of the basis for this exercise, see Chapter 3, "A Yoga of Healing." It is suggested that you read the following instructions into a tape recorder at a pace that is comfortable. At a later time replay the tape and follow the directions.

This exercise is intended to be used with other techniques for self-healing of cases of repetitive habit patterns, recurring fears or anxieties, or a persistent sense of depression. The underlying assumption is that in a state of health, emotions are energy patterns in a constant, unimpeded flow. The task is to reaffirm this holomovement within one's psychodynamic field and to consciously assist in its repatterning.

1. Sit in a comfortable position and quietly center yourself; that is, ignore any outside distractions and gently allow your mind to consider only thoughts that have to do with your innermost self.

2. Breathe quietly at your normal rate. Allow the emotion or the thought you want to deal with to arise to consciousness. Do not be afraid of it; simply recognize its presence.

Note: This exercise can be done as often as time permits, preferably at least twice a day when you have a few moments to yourself, such as when awakening in the morning and just before you fall asleep at night.

You will find that in time you will be able to recall the buoyancy and high energy of these joyous feeling tones upon demand. As you allow them deeper expression, the memory of the experience will nurture you throughout the day. Allow the experience to grow on its own terms; that is, don't try to program it, and it will nurture you in its own way.

3. At the next exhalation, use the outward movement of your breath to direct the thought or emotion outward toward the periphery of your field, just beyond the boundary of your skin.

4. Center yourself once again. When you feel that sense of quietude, call up to your imagination a memory of a time of joyousness in your life. Try to imagine yourself in that situation once again and sense the spontaneous feeling of that moment of rejoicing.

5. Allow joy to permeate through you so that you have a sense of lightness and buoyancy. However, do not hold on to the energy of this experience; let it flow freely outward toward the periphery of your field.

6. If you find that the flow is impeded by knots of tension, allow this sense of elation to flow into and around this stressed complex. Bathe it in the joyous and uplifting energy, and then direct these feeling tones toward the outermost reaches of your psychodynamic field.

APPENDIX F

Vivid Visualization: Review of the Literature and Theoretical Rationale

Visualization is an introspective act that is fundamental to primary human thought processes, such as memory, problem solving, and goal setting. Visualization appears to develop during the first year of life as the child increasingly engages in oculomotor coordination, hand-eye coordination, and locomotion. As the child experiences the reality of objects and gains a measure of control over that reality, it is thought that the child concomitantly learns to form concepts about those objects in some internal manner.[90] However, it is not yet fully understood *how* concept formation creates "pictures in the brain" so that one thereafter recognizes a class of objects whether they are objectively present or whether only the symbol of the object is perceived. Neither is it understood how one conjures up mental images at will.

Currently, the most vigorous study of visualization arises from research into eidetic imagery, which is concerned with vivid mental images, and its relation to learning theory,[91] with clarity of image and creative self-perception,[92] and with hypnotic susceptability.[93] The combined use of visualization and relaxation procedures in autogenic training[94] and in biofeedback,[95] both of which are based on autosuggestion, have been found to elicit profound physiological effects. Simonton, Matthew-Simonton, and Creighton have demonstrated that the use of visualization techniques with methods of stress reduction can also significantly affect the development of cancers in selected patients.[96] Achterberg and Lawton (see Chapter 5, note 82) have developed an instrument, IMAGE-CA, that formalizes imagery drawings of patients with cancer so that objective scoring and statistical predictions are made possible. Visualization as perception, therefore, is a measurable variable.

Visualization, however, has not been conclusively studied as an intrapsychic event. From a neurological point of view it has been suggested—but never verified—that the same kind of biological synthesis that occurs within the neurological substrata of the visual tracts underlies both visualization as an interior process and visualization as an objective perception. However, in the latter instance this synthesis is put into effect by visual information from the external environment, but in the former case the visualization is based on stored information.[97] Visualization as an intrapsychic event, therefore, is analyzed and interpreted within a neurological and psychological context.

A special case of intrapsychic visualization is the apparently supranormal, vivid visualizations in which there is neither stored information about the object nor about incidents in the subject's environmental surround. Nevertheless, the information received in this supranormal manner upon examination proves to be correct. The most famous incident in recent history about which there is valid historical record occurred in the eighteenth century to Emmanuel Swedenborg.[98] The incident took place at a party in Paris. During the party Swedenborg became visibly alarmed. When he was asked what was the matter, he said that a large fire was occurring at that time near his home in Stockholm. He went on to describe the fire in detail. Several days later, when the mail boat came into port, his account was confirmed.

Anecdotal records abound, but not until Rhine, Rhine, and Pratt of Duke University began to study paranormal perception within a controlled research frame that lent itself to statistical analysis was the study of paranormal perception given serious attention in the behavioral sciences.[99,100] Their studies were essentially based on card guessing, but they offered a structured, controlled way by which the ability to perceive an object at an unusual distance could be tested. Soal, an English mathematician, undertook independent research of a similar nature.[101] Many of Rhine's and Soal's experiments were conducted so that persons who had access to the cards were at a considerable distance from the subject who was trying to perceive the card. In both Rhine's and Soal's studies the subjects were in a fully conscious and alert state.

For many years the statistical studies of Rhine and Soal dominated the research on perception at a distance by paranormal means, so that the study protocol became standardized. The more human aspects of this process did not lend themselves to acceptable research precedures until the early 1960s. One of the first researchers to search out physiological correlates of paranormal perception was Dean.[102] With the use of an instrument called a plethysmograph, measurements could be taken on changes in the blood volume of a subject's finger while that subject was attempting to receive information telepathically from a person not in the same room. At the time of this experiment, changes in blood volume were thought to be valid indicators of changes in the autonomic nervous system functioning; today biofeedback research has demonstrated that volitional control (by use of will power and imagery) can intervene.[103]

Dean's procedure was to randomly select names from a telephone directory and put them on target cards. On another group of cards were names that were well known to the subject (the Receiver). Both samples of cards were pooled and mixed. Another person (the Transmitter), who was stationed at a considerable distance from the Receiver, randomly selected one card at a time from the combined deck of cards and looked at each selected card one at a time for a specified length of time. Dean found significant differences in the blood volume in the fingers of the Receivers when the Transmitter looked at a name well known to the Receiver, as compared with the Receiver's plethysmographic measurements when the Transmitter looked at a randomly selected name.

Tart (see Chapter 5, note 75) and Doyd[104] also used physiological variables to test correlates of this telepathic mode of perception, which was named psi cognition. A Receiver was placed in an electrically protected room, such as a Faraday cage; the Receiver's electroencephalographic (EEG) tracings were recorded. Simultaneously in a second room some distance from the first, another person—the Transmitter—was stimulated at random intervals. The time of each stimulation was automatically recorded on the Receiver's EEG record without his or her knowledge.

In Tart's study the Transmitter was stimulated by electric shock. Doyd asked his Transmitters to think of a red triangle each time a red light flashed on. Tart found that the Receivers had a significant reduction in amplitude and a desynchronization of alpha waves when their Transmitters were electrically stimulated. Doyd noted a consistent evoked potential in his Receivers upon the presentation of the stimulus (the red light flash) to their Transmitters. Inferences of these physiological changes were not discussed.

Building upon these studies, Targ and Puthoff tested for non-cognitive awareness of events occurring at a place remote from where the Receiver was stationed (See Chapter 5, notes 76 and 77). Using a research design similar to that of Tart and Doyd, they had two subjects separated from each other in different rooms. Each of the rooms was shielded from both sound and electric stimuli. The subjects were connected to an EEG apparatus. Targ and Puthoff hypothesized that there would be a correlation between the EEG alpha activity of both subjects when one subject was stimulated; that is, upon stimulation of one subject, there would be a coupling effect or a reflection of the alpha readings of the second subject, even though the two subjects were in different rooms. In this case it could be thought that the first subject would be acting as a Transmitter and the second as a Receiver. A remotely controlled stroboscopic light flash was used as a stimulus to the Transmitter. Appropriate controls were instituted to monitor whether the research findings might be influenced by system artifacts of the research design, electromagnetic pickup between the machines, or subtle unconscious cueing by members of the research team.

Seven runs of thirty-six trials, each of which lasted ten seconds, were done. The Receiver's alpha activity record demonstrated a significant reduction in both average power ($p < .04$) and peak power ($p < .03$) upon stroboscopic flash stimulation as compared with no-flash data. The reduction in amplitude and desynchronization of alpha, which would indicate an arousal response, was similar to Tart's findings noted above.

Targ and Puthoff conducted continued descriptive research on the ability of individuals to be aware of events occurring at a distance. They termed this mode of perception "remote viewing." Specifically, this term refers to the ability of some individuals to gain access to information that usually is not normally perceptible and to correctly describe this information. The underlying dynamics of this manner of information transfer are admittedly not clear either neurophysiologically or psychologically at this time.

These investigators reported on fifty-one laboratory-controlled double-blind experiments with nine subjects who had previous opportunities to develop remote perceptual abilities. These subjects acted as Receivers; the investigators themselves acted as the Transmitters.

The experiments were set up so that a Transmitter was sent under sealed orders to a remote geographical location at a specified time. The locations were chosen without the knowledge of the investigators by a person who was not connected with the experiment. While at the location the Transmitter kept a detailed record of the geographical setting and also took photographs of the landscape, buildings, and other objects within his or her line of vision. Simultaneously the Receiver, who was seated with an uninformed observer in the laboratory, either drew or wrote a description of his or her perceptions of the geographical setting in which the Transmitter was at a specified time. This written material was evaluated for rank order against the verbal or pictorial records of the Transmitter by a research analyst not involved in the study. The statistical analysis for the sum of ranks greatly exceeded expectations. The report cites the confidence interval for each of the subjects.

The investigators reported three principal findings:

1. It is possible to obtain significant amounts of accurate information from remote locations.

2. An increase in the distance from a few meters up to 4,000 kilometers separating the subject from the scene does not in any apparent way degrade the quality or the accuracy of perceptions.

3. The use of Faraday cage electric shielding does not prevent high-quality descriptions from being obtained.

SUMMARY

In summary, therefore, paranormal ability to perceive correctly over long distances has strong statistical as well as descriptive support. Certain autonomic nervous system changes, such as finger blood volume, can occur in the Receiver when a Transmitter is perceiving information about a person known to the Receiver. Predictable EEG changes occur in a Receiver when a Transmitter is electrically shocked, when a Transmitter looks at a specific image, or when a Transmitter experiences a photic driving (by strobe light stimulus) of his or her own brain waves. Finally, detailed descriptions about remote locations can be accurately transmitted by persons at a site to other persons at a distance. In this case, the amount of distance separating the Receiver from the site does not interfere with either the quality or the accuracy of the perceptions, nor is the caliber of the descriptions affected by electric shielding of the Receiver.

CRITICAL REVIEWS

Recent research findings on biofeedback have demonstrated that there can be volitional control over autonomic nervous system functioning, as noted above in reference to the Dean study on finger blood volume (although it was not known at the time of that study). It should also be noted that the Targ and Puthoff study has met with criticism and reservations. Ornstein considers this study as "tentative and investigative . . . interesting pilot studies."[105] A *Scientific American* editorial reported on the *post hoc* examination of five unpublished transcripts in the Targ and Puthoff data by Marks and Kamman of the University of Otago in New Zealand (See Chapter 5, note 78). They were able to find "cues in each of them revealing the transcript's position in the sequence" in which the data was presented to the Receiver. These cues, Marks and Kamman claim, enabled them "to match each of the five transcripts with the proper site—without ever having visited the site!" They do not remark, however, on the validity of the subjects' ability. As noted in the body of this report, the writer took precautions to control for such inadvertent cueing in her research on Vivid Visualization.

THEORETICAL RATIONALE

A review of the literature would indicate that the basis of a Receiver's awareness of the information transfer is neurological since both autonomic nervous system and central nervous system (via EEG recordings) indices have been reported. The finding that distance does not interfere with the accuracy of the information transmitted to the Receiver, however, does not suggest a simple rationale. This finding does not fit the current understanding of the structure of space as it relates to man, that is, with the principle of the inverse square ratio, in which an effect will predictably decrease in proportion to the distance it travels. This anomaly, or seeming paradox, indicates a need to reexamine the present model.

Vivid Visualization: Statistical Analysis

Hypothesis 1: The data from the three small groups were independent measures. The individual members of each group were different, and the groups were studied at different times, although the protocol for all the groups was the same. The data on the factors of Hits, Misses, and Items Not Perceived were treated in two different ways:

1. The three small groups were tested by multiple t tests to determine whether there were any significant differences between the means of the Hits, Misses, and Items Not Perceived, and

2. An analysis of variance was done to determine if there was any significant interaction in reference to these measures.

It was found that there was no significant difference either between the means of the three small groups (Table 5) or in their interaction (Tables 6, 7, and 8). Therefore, the data were then collapsed into one larger sample, which then became the Experimental Group tested in Hypotheses 2 to 5.

Hypothesis 2: A Fisher's t test for uncorrelated means was done between the means of the criterion measures in the collapsed experimental sample (Experimental Group) and the Control Group (Tables 9 and 10). The Fisher's t was equal to 5.46 at 52 degrees of freedom, $p < .001$, which supported Hypothesis 2.

Hypothesis 3: This hypothesis was confirmed at the .001 level of confidence when a Fisher's t for uncorrelated means was em-

TABLE 5
Multiple Fisher's *t* Tests Re: Differences Between the
Uncorrelated Means of Data on Perceptions of the Three
Experimental Small Groups

Source	N	E	$\bar{x}$	Ex²	SD	Fishers *t*	Significance @ 13 df
Hits:							
Group 1	10	88	8.8	137.2	3.70		
Group 2	10	72	7.2	65.7	2.56		
Group 3	10	66	6.6	116.4	3.41		
$\bar{x}_I \times \bar{x}_{II}$						1.07	n.s.
$\bar{x}_{II} \times \bar{x}_{III}$						0.42	n.s.
$\bar{x}_I \times \bar{x}_{III}$						1.31	n.s.
Misses:							
Group 1	10	16	1.6	22.4	1.50		
Group 2	10	7	0.7	10.1	1.004		
Group 3	10	10	1.0	10.0	1.0		
$\bar{x}_I \times \bar{x}_{II}$						1.5	n.s.
$\bar{x}_{II} \times \bar{x}_{III}$						0.638	n.s.
$\bar{x}_I \times \bar{x}_{III}$						1.0	n.s.
Not Perceived							
Group 1	10	28	2.8	15.6	1.25		
Group 2	10	22	2.2	11.6	1.08		
Group 3	10	19	1.9	18.9	1.37		
$\bar{x}_I \times \bar{x}_{II}$						1.09	n.s.
$\bar{x}_{II} \times \bar{x}_{III}$						0.52	n.s.
$\bar{x}_I \times \bar{x}_{III}$						1.45	n.s.

ployed. The difference between the mean of the Misses in the Experimental Group and that of the Control Group was 7.83. At 52 degrees of freedom, $p < .001$ in support of this hypothesis also.

Hypothesis 4: A Fisher's *t* for uncorrelated means supported Hypothesis 4. In this case the difference between the means of Items Not Perceived in the Experimental Group and the similar means in the Control Group demonstrated a Fisher's *t* of 25.8: 52 degrees of freedom, $p < .001$. Table 8 illustrates that the data for Hypotheses 2, 3, and 4 were all in the predicted direction.

TABLE 6
Analysis of Variance of Data on Hits in the Three Experimental Small Groups and F Ratios

Source	Sum of Squares	Degrees of Freedom	Estimate of Variance	F Ratio
Between Rows (Group 1)	25.9	2	12.95	1.33 n.s.
Between Columns (Healer A/B)	10.8	1	10.8	1.11 n.s.
Interaction	2.4	2	1.2	0.12 n.s.
Within Sets	234.4	24	9.77	
Total	273.5	29		
Between Sets	39.1			

TABLE 7
Analysis of Variance of Data on Misses in the Three Experimental Small Groups and F Ratios

Source	Sum of Squares	Degrees of Freedom	Estimate of Variance	F Ratio
Between Rows	4.2	2	2.1	1.25 n.s.
Between Columns	0	1	0	xx
Interaction	2.1	2	1.05	0.63 n.s.
Within Sets	40.4	24	1.68	
Total	46.7	29		
Between Sets	6.3			

Hypothesis 5: The hypothesis was intended to indicate whether there had been consistency in the ability of the Nurse-Meditators in the Experimental Group to have equable variations in their Vivid Visualizations of both Patients assigned to each team. For this purpose Pearson's product-moment coefficient of correlation between their perceptions of their first Patient and their second Patient on the measures Hits, Misses, and Items Not Perceived was done on the fifteen pairs of Patients in the Experimental Group. A t ratio

TABLE 8

Analysis of Variance of Data on Items Not Perceived in the
Three Experimental Small Groups and F Ratios

Source	Sum of Squares	Degrees of Freedom	Estimate of Variance	F Ratio
Between Rows	4.2	2	2.1	1.19 n.s.
Between Columns	0.8	1	0.8	0.45 n.s.
Interaction	2.9	2	1.45	0.82 n.s.
Within Sets	42.4	24	1.77	
Total	50.3	29		
Between Sets	7.9			

TABLE 9

Fisher's t for Testing a Difference Between Uncorrelated
Means of Experimental Group as a Whole and the Control
Group on Hits, Misses, and Items Not Perceived*

	Hits	Misses	Not Perceived
Fisher's t	5.46**	7.83**	25.8**

*$df = 52$
**$- p < .001$

TABLE 10

Means and Standard Deviations for Hits, Misses, and Items
Not Perceived for Experimental Group as a Whole and the
Control Group

	Experimental (N = 30)			Control (N = 24)		
	Hits	Misses	Not Perceived	Hits	Misses	Not Perceived
$\bar{x}$:	7.5	1.1	2.3	3.3	6.9	12.2
Ex^2:	345.5	46.7	50.3	64.96	333.84	52.36
σ:	3.39	1.25	1.29	1.65	3.73	1.48
$\acute{6}$:	0.44	0.16	0.17	0.24	0.48	0.19

TABLE 11
Pearson's Product Moment Coefficient of Correlation
of Patient #1 and Patient #2 in the Experimental Group
on the Measures of Hits, Misses, and Items Not Perceived,
and t Ratio for Testing the Significance of Each Coefficient
of Correlation*

	Pearson's $r_{1,2}$	t Ratio	Level of Confidence
Hits	.76	4.2	$p < .01$
Misses	.75	4.1	$p < .01$
Not Perceived	.56	2.4	$p < .05$

*Degrees of freedom: 13
 N = 15 pairs

for determining the level of confidence of each coefficient of correlation also was done. All data are enumerated in Table 11.

A marked relationship, or high correlation, is noted for both the Hits ($r = .76$) and Misses ($r = .75$), in both of these cases at 13 degrees of freedom, $p < .01$. On the measure of Items Not Perceived, there is a substantive relationship noted for this moderate correlation which, however, is significant at 13 degrees of freedom, $p < .05$.

Vivid Visualization: Nurse-Meditator's Form

INSTRUCTIONS:

*E*nclosed please find the names of two persons who are ill, each of whom we would like you to think of for three consecutive days at these stipulated times each day: _____. The time you spend thinking of each healee is limited only by your individual judgment; it is suggested, however, that both the healing and the writing of notes on each healee should take no more than one half-hour on each of the three days. Please think of the healee in the following manner:

1. Center (meditation can be done either before or after this exercise).

2. When you feel you are on center, think of the healee by name.

3. Try to visualize the healee.

4. Visualize yourself in the vicinity of the healee.

5. Note the condition of the healee and his or her environment.

6. Decide how you can best help the healee in his present condition.

7. Think therapeutically of the healee, as if you are actually doing Therapeutic Touch.

8. At end of healing, take a moment to register a judgment on how well the healing attempt succeeded before going on to the next healee.

9. Come back to center before terminating this exercise and review impressions.

10. Fill out a form for your experience with each healee each day. Keep a carbon copy, if you wish, for your own records. Send the original to Principal Investigator each day in the envelopes provided.

We thank you very much for taking part in this study. There is little that is known in our culture about these phenomena, and we hope that this study will provide some useful insights. Should this occur, it will be due to the volunteer efforts of yourself and others who will have helped to push back a bit the veils of ignorance that still persist in our time.

Healer: _____   Date: _____

Healee: _____   Time of Healing: _____ to _____

Note any medications and/or vitamins healer is taking:

_____

Personal biorhythm data of healer:

Time of

Meals: Breakfast _____   Lunch _____   Supper _____

Were snacks taken? _____   Time of day _____

Sleep time on previous night: _____ to _____

Day of menstrual cycle: _____

Today's phase of the moon: _____

General weather conditions (include barometric pressure reading):

_____

Personal physiological data before and after healings:

	Pulse	Respiration	Temperature	B/P, if possible
Before Healing:	_____	_____	_____	_____
After Healing:	_____	_____	_____	_____

Brief resume of meditation content: _____

_____

_____

_____

Description of the healing experience (use more space as needed, draw if necessary)

Imagery _____

_____

Impression (include indication of intensity): _____

_____

Symbols: _____

_____

Specific visualizations: _____

_____

_____

_____

Personal physical or emotional sensations: _____

_____

_____

Physical or emotional sensations that seem to be related to the healee:

_____

_____

_____

Colors, sounds, odors, or other sensations noted during the healing experience: _____

_____

_____

_____

Description of what the healer thought happened to the healee during the healing experience: _____

_____

_____

_____

_____

Impressions relative to the physical environment of the healee (draw if possible): _____

_____

_____

Impressions relative to the healee's physical and emotional state, thoughts, and/or interactions with others:

_____

_____

_____

_____

_____

Judgment on how well the healing attempt succeeded: _____

_____

_____

Miscellaneous comments:

APPENDIX I

Vivid Visualization: Nurse-Observer's Form

INSTRUCTIONS:

*E*nclosed please find the forms we would like you to fill in on each of the two patients you have volunteered to observe for three consecutive days at the stipulated times, and addressed, stamped envelopes. We would like you to observe each patient for five minutes twice during the following time _____ on each of the three days, and for five minutes in the hour previous to this, e.g., _____ and for five minutes in the hour following this time, e.g., _____ each day. It is to be understood that you have obtained permission from the patient and the health facility to make these observations.

Jot down notes unobtrusively during these times and then fill out one form for each patient each day, enclose them in one of the addressed envelopes that are attached, and mail them each day to the Investigator.

Should you wish to observe the patient at additional times, this would be much appreciated; however, we would like the information noted at the specific times stated above. Please make yourself familiar with the form before you begin your observations so that you will be aware of the significant kinds of information we are seeking. Do not hesitate to add other information that you think might be useful.

Fill out one form on your observations of each patient each day. Keep a carbon copy, if you wish, for your own records.

PROTOCOL FOR INFORMING THE HEALTH FACILITY ABOUT THE STUDY

It is requested that you get the permission of the attending physician, the Department of Nursing, and the health facility's research review board, if the facility requires it, before starting this study. It is suggested that they be told that you would like to participate in observing the effects other persons' thoughts and impressions might have on patients.

PROTOCOL FOR INFORMING THE PATIENT ABOUT THE STUDY

It is suggested that you tell the patient that you are participating in a study in which your observation of patients' conditions will be checked against the observations of other nurses. It is *not* suggested that you go into any other details of the study until the study period has been completed; however, the patient's consent should be obtained verbally or in writing.

We thank you very much for taking part in this study. There is little that is known in our culture about these phenomena, and we hope that this study will provide some useful insights. Should this occur, it will be due to the volunteer efforts of yourself and others who will have helped to push back a bit the veils of ignorance that still persist in our time.

Observer: _____ Date: _____

Patient: _____ Sex:_____ Age: _____ Level of Education:

1. Medical Diagnosis: _____

   _____

2. Nursing Assessment: _____

   _____

3. Brief case history: _____

_____

_____

_____

4. Significant laboratory findings: _____

_____

5. General description of the health facility: _____

_____

6. Specific description of patient's room (draw diagram):

7. People who are significant to the patient: _____

_____

8. What is the patient's physical condition and level of awareness?

Time: _____

_____

_____

Time: _____

_____

_____

Time: _____

_____

_____

9. How does the patient feel? (subjective symptoms)

Time: _____

_____

_____

Time: _____

_____

_____

Time: _____

_____

_____

10. Do you have any particular impressions about the patient's condition?

Time: _____

_____

_____

Time: _____

_____

_____

Time: _____

_____

_____

11. Were any dreams related by the patient?

Time: _____

_____

_____

Time: _____

_____

_____

Time: _____

_____

_____

12. Did the patient relate any other subjective impressions?

    Time: _____

    _____

    _____

    Time: _____

    _____

    _____

    Time: _____

    _____

    _____

13. What were the activities and interactions (with patients, staff, relatives, etc.) of the patient?

    Time: _____

    _____

    _____

    Time: _____

    _____

    _____

    Time: _____

    _____

    _____

14. Were there other occurrences of note that happened to the patient?

    Time: _____

    _____

    _____

    Time: _____

    _____

    _____

Time: _____

_____

_____

15. Are there further significant observations? (e.g., what was pa-
    tient and persons who interacted with the patient wearing, what
    did they talk about, what seemed to be the emotional tone,
    etc.)

    Time: _____

    _____

    _____

    Time: _____

    _____

    _____

    Time: _____

    _____

    _____

16. What are your impressions about any part of this experience?
    Please feel free to write fully.

    ─────────

Note: Items 1–7 need only be noted on Day 1 unless there is a change in
the patient's condition, relations, or location.

APPENDIX J

Therapeutic Touch During Childbirth Preparation by the Lamaze Method and its Relation to Marital Satisfaction and State Anxiety of the Married Couple*

INTRODUCTION

One of the most frightening traditional assumptions in Western culture has been that pain is a natural concomitant of childbirth (see Chapter 7, note 85). This belief has been so ingrained in the cultural mores as to be considered basic in the care of childbearing mothers. The effect of this belief has been to foster an attitude in which the birthing process has been construed to be necessarily painful. However, research within the context of the Pavlovian theory of conditioning-response sets has been done in the U.S.S.R. that has demonstrated that a reflex action conditioned to be painful can purposely, by mindset, be converted into a physiological stimulus that seems painless. A method has been devised to translate this finding into techniques by which the apparent pain of childbirth can be ameliorated. A French obstetrician, Fernand Lamaze, was

*Federal support was given this study through the Nursing Research Emphasis Grant for Doctoral Programs, Department of Health and Human Resources, U.S. Public Health Service. #NU-00833-02, Patricia Winstead-Fry, Ph.D., R.N.. Director. Appreciation for collegial support and critique is expressed to Professors Patricia Winstead-Fry, Carol Hoskins, Patricia Hurley, and Therese Connell-Meehan.

157

able to further develop this technique and adapt it to his native French culture in 1952.[106] Since then it has found acceptance in many countries, particularly in the United States, where it has become known as the Lamaze Method of prepared childbirth.

This method is essentially concerned with the education and conditioning of the mother's reflexes during the last trimester of pregnancy. The conditioning is done by specific verbal commands given by a partner or by the father of the child. These commands are theorized to divert the mother's attention from any discomfort brought on by the physical exertion during labor and to thereby inhibit the sympathetic spread of autonomic nervous system "flight" reactions. In this way she can actively and painlessly participate in the regulation of her own labor. Verbal commands are used as a method of internal signaling. The words are specific for each stage of labor and delivery; they act as the conditioning stimuli for the mother's efforts during birthing.[107]

The Lamaze Method has met with considerable success; however, it is a mother-centered process. The father of the child is relegated to the sidelines to act out the role of "coach." He cues the mother to the appropriate efforts. He doubles as a cheering section to encourage her during the process. His involvement in the birthing process is vicarious, an empathic participation at best. For the father there is no active link with the birthing event except for the act of conception. The delivery process, like the process of pregnancy, is a primal experience for the mother only. This is a cultural limitation (there are cultures that allow the father to act out birth pains) that can foster a negative climate for the father's conscious realization and development of the contrasexual element of his psyche, the anima. This psychological factor is known to precondition attitudes and behaviors that are concerned with family-centered relationships.

The present study proposed to confront this cultural limitation by actively engaging the father in the pregnancy and in the birthing process of his child through the medium of Therapeutic Touch. In so involving the father while he also plays the role of coach to the mother, it was expected that family-centered psychodynamics, such as the fulfillment of emotional and interactional needs by the marital partners and their anxiety, would be enhanced in significant measure beyond similar relationships developed by couples engaged only in the Lamaze Method.

Therapeutic Touch During Childbirth Preparation: Definition of Terms

THERAPEUTIC TOUCH

*T*heoretically, Therapeutic Touch is defined for the purposes of this study as a treatment wherein the husband:

1. Centers himself in an act of interior self-relatedness and becomes aware of himself as an open system of energies in constant flux.

2. Makes a strong mental intention to therapeutically support his wife in the maintenance of optimum health.

3. Moves his hands about two to four inches away from his wife's body, palms towards the body surface, and slowly but steadily moves them in a head-to-feet direction, meanwhile attuning his senses to the condition of his wife's energy field by becoming aware of sensory cues in his hands.

4. Redirects any felt tension in his wife's energy field by movement of his hands.

5. Concentrates his attention on the specific direction and modulation of these energies and expresses this direction or modulation of energy through the nature of the movements of his hands within his wife's energy field.

6. Keeps his hands now in the area of his wife's solar plexus, either in body contact or up to four inches away from her body surface (a subjective decision). This area is in the front of the body at about the level of the waist, just above the umbilicus.

159

7. Leaves his hands so placed for no longer than five minutes. The total time of the treatment is no longer than ten minutes (See Chapter 1, note 12).

Operationally, Therapeutic Touch is defined as a score of at least thirty on the Subjective Experience of Therapeutic Touch Scale (SETTS). SETTS is a Likert-type scale that was tested originally by Fry and Krieger on a national sample of 250 professional persons who practiced Therapeutic Touch; this test has been independently replicated by Ferguson. (See Chapter 1, note 25.) SETTS[108] can distinguish between three levels of practitioners at the .0001 level of confidence.[109] (See Appendix R.)

CHILDBIRTH PREPARATION BY THE LAMAZE METHOD

In the Lamaze Method an expectant couple attends a series of classes whose purpose is to prepare pregnant women for labor and delivery of their children. The focus of these classes is on the development of conditioned reflexes in response to uterine contractions. The method involves specific training to ensure conscious, active participation by the woman in labor to cope with the stress of childbirth.

FAMILY-CENTERED PSYCHODYNAMIC RELATIONSHIPS

These are construed as being based on marital satisfaction and are demonstrated in the level of state anxiety.

Marital satisfaction refers to feelings of happiness and satisfaction within the marital unit that are expressed by the marriage partners. Marital satisfaction is measured by the Interpersonal Conflict Scale (ICS) as developed by Hoskins and Merrifield.[110]

State anxiety refers to a transitory emotional state that is characterized by subjective, consciously perceived feelings of tension and apprehension accompanied by intensified autonomic nervous system activity. State anxiety is measured by the Self-Evaluation Questionnaire, STAI Form X-1, as developed by Spielberger, Gorsuch and Lushene.[111]

Therapeutic Touch During Childbirth Preparation: Delimitations of the Study, Hypotheses, and Research Question

DELIMITATIONS

1. Limited to married couples who participated in Lamaze classes for at least four sessions.

2. Mothers were primaparous (pregnant for the first time) and had an uncomplicated prenatal experience; the child was vaginally delivered, and it was a normal newborn.

3. All couples were married at the time of conception.

4. Since all the measuring tools require a comprehension of English, only English-speaking persons made up the study sample.

GENERAL HYPOTHESIS

Practice of Therapeutic Touch by husbands on their primaparous wives during childbirth preparation will enhance their family-centered psychodynamic relationships.

SUBHYPOTHESES

1. Controlling for differences in level of marital satisfaction at antepartum, couples who engage in Therapeutic Touch and prepared childbirth will demonstrate greater marital satisfaction at post-partum than couples who only use prepared childbirth.

2. Controlling for differences in state anxiety at antepartum, couples who engage in Therapeutic Touch and prepared childbirth will demonstrate a decreased level of state anxiety at postpartum when compared to couples who use only prepared childbirth.

RESEARCH QUESTION

Is there a differential effect among the subjects' scores on the various behavioral facets of the Interpersonal Conflict Scale in this sample?

Therapeutic Touch During Childbirth Preparation: Significance of the Study

*T*his study seeks to validate the use of Therapeutic Touch as an adjunct to childbirth preparation by the Lamaze Method in enhancing marital satisfaction and by simultaneously decreasing state anxiety. Fathers with this skill are able to offer their wives another source of comfort during the pregnancy. By reducing anxiety, it is conceivable that Therapeutic Touch could have beneficial effects on the physiological functioning of newborns, on the maternal use of analgesics, and on the husband's attitudes toward his involvement in the birthing process. In contributing to an increase in marital satisfaction, the practice of Therapeutic Touch could contribute to deeper bonding of the married couple with each other and with their child and provide a model for caring and concern for others within their sphere of influence; possibly it could also elicit other positive nonverbal behavior between spouses and within the family.

APPENDIX N

Therapeutic Touch During Childbirth Preparation: Review of the Literature

This study brings together two methods of pain reduction, Therapeutic Touch and the Lamaze method of prepared childbirth. It seeks to establish their relationship to two parameters of family interaction; specifically, to marital satisfaction and state anxiety. The logic of this inquiry is demonstrated in the following brief review and critique of research related to the variables under study.

THERAPEUTIC TOUCH

Therapeutic Touch was first described by Krieger in 1972. It is an act of healing or helping that derives from the laying-on of hands; however, unlike traditional laying-on of hands, Therapeutic Touch is not done within a religious context, nor is the healing or helping that occurs considered to be a function of the faith of the healer and/or the client (see Chapter 1, note 17).

Therapeutic Touch is known to produce a state of deep relaxation in the client (see Chapter 1, note 22 and Chapter 3, note 44). Further, it is a highly personalized interaction (see Chapter 1, note 12); clients report feelings of deep caring, empathy, and emotional support from the Therapeutic Touch practitioner.

With regard to the dependent variables in this study—marital satisfaction and state anxiety—there are no research data at this time on the interaction or relationship of marital satisfaction and Therapeutic Touch. However, there is a sound theoretical link drawn from family systems theory. Family therapists hypothesize that the level of anxiety in a family system is the basic determinant of the quality of a marriage (Bowen). Therapeutic Touch is known to decrease anxiety in clinical studies (see Chapter 1, note 12), and this relationship has been supported in two doctoral studies (see Chapter 1, notes 19 and 21). It is logical, therefore, to hypothesize that Therapeutic Touch will enhance marital satisfaction by decreasing state anxiety.

This study will extend the literature dealing with Therapeutic Touch and anxiety by examining a different population, specifically childbearing couples. Both Heidt and Quinn studied the effects of Therapeutic Touch in reducing anxiety in hospitalized cardiovascular patients. Both studies documented statistically significant decreases in state anxiety ($p < .01$) in their experimental groups, which were treated with Therapeutic Touch, when compared to control groups having no touch or casual touch.

PREPARED CHILDBIRTH

The relationship of prepared childbirth to marital satisfaction and state anxiety is complex and confusing. The central objective of prepared childbirth is to reduce the fear-tension-pain syndrome through conditioned response. Dick-Read perceives anxiety as the precursor of the syndrome. He states, "Unless her [the mother in labor] anxiety is alleviated, the fear-tension-pain syndrome cycle is put into motion because of the stimulation of the sympathetic nervous system."

Research has not always supported this contention, however. Huttel, Mitehill, Fisher, and Meyer (1972), as well as Zak, Someroff, and Farnum (1975), have found no relationship between anxiety reduction and the Lamaze Method of Childbirth Preparation. Other authors claim such a relationship, although most of this latter literature is concerned with decreased anxiety and the ability to conceive and carry a pregnancy (Crandon 1979; Lederman, Lederman, Work, and McCann 1979). Studies on the relationship of attendence at desensitization classes and the use of the Lamaze Method was done by Beck, Siegel, Davidson, Kormeir, Breitenstein, and Hall 1980 and by Kondas, and Seitnicks 1972. Desensitization refers to various stress-reduction methods. Although the content of the reports is based on clinical data that are not entirely clear and the conclusions are not in direct agreement, they nevertheless do serve to add clinical justification for the linking of Therapeutic Touch and the Lamaze method of prepared childbirth. In further support of this proposal, it could be stated that one result of Therapeutic Touch that has been clinically verified is a significant relaxation response in the healee, or client. This response is posited for desensitization as well. In reference to Therapeutic Touch, the substantive finding that justified the description of relaxation response was characterized by decreased anxiety, more relaxed breathing patterns (that is, deeper, slower respirations), decreased heart rate, and increased alpha and theta brain-wave activity (see Chapter 1, notes 17 and 22).

In reference to the interaction between prepared childbirth and marital satisfaction, the findings are also obscure. Claims have been made that prepared childbirth increases marital satisfaction; however, the bases of these claims are either methodologically flawed research or verbal testimony. The most common flaws noted are lack of control groups, retrospective recall of predelivery events, lack of reliability and validity in the measurement tools, and "overgeneralizations based on minimal statistical analysis."[112]

Moore designed a doctoral dissertation whose objective was to bring rigorous empirical inquiry to the question of marital satisfaction and prepared childbirth. She used a longitudinal design and found that husbands' level of marital satisfaction increases after prepared childbirth classes but that the wives' scores do not increase. This effect was particularly noted on the emotional factor of the instrument. Moore noted more of a change in the second factor, the interaction factor, of the instrument, but this was not statistically significant. This she attributed to the husbands' role in the Lamaze method. The husband, she noted, is a "coach." He and the wife talk about the labor; they work toward a common goal, and on that level they share the birth experience. This role essentially is instrumental for the husband, but it does not necessarily involve empathy or other deep emotional components. A good coach could in fact be emotionally detached. In designing the present study, the inclusion of Therapeutic Touch was conceived as a mode of highly personalized interaction that would act to enhance the emotional connectedness of the couple.

APPENDIX O

Therapeutic Touch During Childbirth Preparation: Methodology, Research Findings, and Discussion

RESEARCH DESIGN

This study was a longitudinal design with generally randomized experimental and control groups. Assignment of subjects was done in a random manner through the selection of the Lamaze teachers who had volunteered to assist in this study. After random selection, one class of each Lamaze teacher contributed subjects for the Experimental Group, and a second class of that same teacher contributed subjects for the Control Group. Selection was continued in this manner until forty couples who met the delimitations of this study were in each group. The number was used to provide for an expected 25-percent attrition rate due to caesarean birth rather than the vaginal birth defined for this study sample. Taking subjects from the same teacher for both the Control and the Experimental groups assured similar learning experiences in each group. The sample consisted of middle-class couples in New York, New Jersey, and Pennsylvania. Since Moore did not find any statistical differences between her Antepartum I Group, early in the antepartum period, and her Antepartum II Group, later in the antepartum period, the pretest for this study was done only once during the antepartum period.

THE SAMPLE

The sample consisted of married couples drawn from the hospital classes or classes taught by the American Society for Psychoprophylaxis in Obstetrics–certified teachers. Efforts were made to en-

167

sure an equal number of hospital-prepared and the Society's prepared couples. However, Moore's findings, noted above, did not find a statistically significant difference between these two methods of childbirth preparation in the prediction of marital satisfaction. Moore's findings, therefore, made this matching less crucial.

Based upon a power of .80, a level of significance of .05 and a moderate effect size, thirty couples were required for each group, the Experimental Group and the Control Group, for a total of sixty married couples in this study. Since the rate for caesarean section in New York City is approximately 25 percent of all deliveries, only couples who had noncomplicated vaginal deliveries and a normal newborn were retained for data analysis. All couples were primaparous, as anxiety is decreased in a second experience with childbirth. Sample characteristics of age, education, and so on were collected on a demographic sheet. Hollingshead's Four Factor Index of Social Status was used to assess social class; all subjects in this study were middle class.

HUMAN SUBJECT PROTECTION ISSUES:

Consent forms for the subjects adhered to New York University Board of Review guidelines for research subjects, and the protocol received Board approval. (See "Explanation Offered to Persons Whose Permission is Requested," Appendix P, and "Consent Form," Appendix Q.)

THE MEASURING TOOLS:

The instruments of this study were the Interpersonal Conflict Scale (ICS), State-Trait Anxiety Inventory (STAI), and the Subjective Experience of Therapeutic Touch Scale (SETTS). The ICS measures "the perceived degree of fulfillment of emotional and interactional needs by the marital partners based upon the perception of these needs" (see Appendix J, note 110). Construct and concurrent validity has been established for the measure and acceptable reliability exists. Moore found reliability coefficients of .83 and .95 for her sample of Lamaze-childbirth-prepared couples, a sample similar to that used in this study (see Appendix N, note 112).

The STAI that was developed by Spielberger, Gorsuch, and Lu-

shene measures two types of anxiety: *state,* or the present, momentary anxiety, and *trait,* the enduring pattern of behaviors accompanying anxiety over time (see Appendix J, note 111). Construct
validity was established for the STAI; also assurance that there is
adequate differentiation between the two anxiety states. Only state
anxiety was measured in this study because labor and delivery are
viewed as producing temporary anxiety. The instrument does not
appear to be affected by repeated measures; in actual clinical use,
repeated usage seems to lead towards greater differentiation among
subjects. It has been utilized with women in labor (Lichella Can-
cheri, Connolly, and Calzolari 1977, and Spielberger and Jacobs 1978).

The SETTS was developed by the research team specifically for
this study (see Appendix K, note 108). It was standardized on a
population of 250 Therapeutic Touch practitioners for the purpose
of quantifying the experience of the healer. Sixty eight self-report
questions make up this Likert-type scale. It was constructed by
deriving questions from authoritative published materials on Therapeutic Touch and from interviews with four recognized experts
who had been practicing Therapeutic Touch for more than five
years. This procedure guaranteed content validity. The test was
administered to a nationwide sample of experienced and less experienced Therapeutic Touch practitioners (n = 250). The alpha
coefficient of reliability was .97. The SETTS distinguishes between
three levels of practitioner at the .0001 level of confidence (See
"Subjective Experience of Therapeutic Touch Scale," Appendix R).

DATA COLLECTION

Estimated time-flow patterns were developed to guide the collection
of data during the research period. In general, the couples completed
their prepared childbirth classes and the fathers were taught Therapeutic Touch by Krieger or her research assistant between the
twenth-fourth and the thirty-sixth week of antepartum. The research
assistant had been previously certified as proficient in both the teaching and practice of Therapeutic Touch. Periods of three to four
consecutive hours were sufficient to teach the basic Therapeutic
Touch techniques to the husbands and to provide time for practice
sessions. During this time there was also a presentation of a videotape prepared especially for this study. The videotape demonstrated

a husband performing Therapeutic Touch on his pregnant wife, in conjunction with the Lamaze techniques. In a voice-over, the principles that had been stated during the teaching period were reiterated (See Appendix S, "Protocol for Teaching Therapeutic Touch to Husbands").

The research assistant and/or Krieger was available to the couples in the Experimental Group for consultation. For this purpose a telephone line was kept available during the weekdays. Further teaching of Therapeutic Touch skills was also available as necessary. Only one couple felt that they needed further supervision, and this was made available to them.

Within one week postpartum, the research assistant telephoned each couple in the entire sample. After assessing that the delimitations of this study had been met (successful vaginal delivery, normal neonate, and so on), arrangements were made for the completion of the posttest materials.

RESULTS AND DISCUSSION

A pretest of the Interpersonal Conflict Scale (ICS) and the State-Trait Anxiety Inventory (STAI) was given to all married couples during the antenatal period to assure equivalency between the Experimental and the Control groups. Table 12 summarizes the data for ICS, and data for STAI is compiled in Table 13.

For the ICS, the Pearson product-moment correlation coefficient was done between the husbands in the two groups and between the wives in both groups. The coefficient between the husbands was $r = 0.67$, for which the t ratio was 4.76. At 28 degrees of freedom, the level of confidence was $p < .01$, which means that if this study were repeated one hundred times, there is less than one chance in those one hundred replications that the results that were obtained were due to random (meaningless) happenings. The correlation between the wives on the ICS was very similar: $r = 0.6$ and the t ratio was 3.96, which also is significant beyond the .01 level of confidence. The data are considered to demonstrate a moderate correlation with substantial relationship and high significance.

The data on the STAI also demonstrated considerable similarity between the wives and between the husbands in the sample. For the husbands the correlation was $r = 0.62$, and the t ratio was

TABLE 12
Analysis of Pretest Scores on the Interpersonal Conflict Scale

	Wives		Husbands	
	Experimental	Control	Experimental	Control
Sum:	1934	1926	2127	2217
Means:	64.5	64.2	70.9	73.9
Standard deviation:	12.1	16.0	14.2	15.4
Pearson correlation coefficient:	$r = 0.6$		$r = 0.67$	
Standard error of r:	$SE_r = 0.12$		$SE_r = 0.102$	
t ratio for correlation coefficient:	$t = 3.96*$		$t = 4.76*$	

*$p < .01$ (df = 28)

TABLE 13
Analysis of Pretest Scores on STAI

	Wives		Husbands	
	Experimental	Control	Experimental	Control
Sum:	908	949	1003	1001
Means:	30.3	31.6	33.4	33.4
Standard deviation:	6.45	7.42	8.24	6.68
Pearson correlation coefficient:	$r = 0.71$		$r = 0.62$	
t ratio for correlation coefficient:	$t = 5.33*$		$t = 4.15*$	

*$p < .01$ (df = 28)

TABLE 14
Analysis of Posttest Scores on the Interpersonal Conflict
Scale

Means experimental:	65.5
Means control:	72.
Number (in either group):	60
Sum of deviations squared (Experimental):	13,923
Sum of deviations squared (Control):	11,524
t ratio $= 2.43*$	

*p $< .05$ (df $= 59$)

4.15. At 28 degrees of freedom, p $< .01$. The correlation between wives was $r = 0.71$, with a t ratio of 5.33, which is significant beyond the .01 level of confidence. The Pearson analysis for the wives was indicative of a high correlation with a marked relationship; the husbands' analysis indicated a more moderate correlation but with a substantial relationship, and both findings had a very high level of statistical significance.

The posttest (postpartum) data are summarized for the ICS in Table 14. There was no significant difference between the means of the Experimental and Control groups on the State-Trait Anxiety Inventory; the means was equal to 30 for each of the groups, with little movement from their pretest scores noted for either group. Implications for these findings will be discussed further on in this appendix.

The ICS tests for perceived lack of fulfillment of marital interaction and emotional needs and is therefore said to indicate level of marital satisfaction. In the Fisher's t test for differences between uncorrelated means in two samples (the Experimental Group and the Control Group) of equal size, the t ratio was 2.43, which, at 59 degrees of freedom, was greater than the .05 level of confidence, as had been hypothesized.

In summary, Hypothesis 1 was statistically supported, whereas the data did not support Hypothesis 2. The ICS has several subsystems in the alternate forms used in this study, and therefore the research question queried which of these subsystems contributed most significantly to the findings. For this purpose a multiple regression was done on the data of these subsystems. However, the results of the regression data did not indicate clear-cut patterns, and therefore a correlation matrix of the data of the subsystems was analyzed. It then was perceived that the very best predictor of marital satisfaction (low interpersonal conflict) in this sample was the subset "Perception of an Other's Feelings," and the next best predictor was the subset "Communications."

In considering the resulting data generated by this study, one can perceive a rationale for the findings. The data on state anxiety will be considered first, and then the findings on marital satisfaction will be discussed.

The research findings relative to Therapeutic Touch and the State-Trait Anxiety Inventory were not similar or supportive of the Heidt (1980)[113] or the Quinn (1982)[114] findings; however, in retrospect the reason calls itself to attention. Before the fact the writer should have recognized that both Heidt's and Quinn's samples were composed of sick people, hospitalized cardiovascular patients who were highly anxious about the cause of their hospitalizations. In contrast, the sample in the present study consisted of normal married couples concerned with a normal, healthy act; pregnancy is not a disease. As noted by the posttest mean of 30 in each of the Groups, state anxiety was quite low and indicated little movement from present scores. In addition, the Lamaze teachers and the Therapeutic Touch research team acted as strong supporters to the married couples. As noted above, the Lamaze teachers contributed subjects to both the Experimental and the Control groups in an attempt to keep the teachers' effect randomized within the sample; nevertheless, one must note the possible effect of support, tacit though it may have been, of the research team on the subjects in the Experimental Group. The possibilities of the latter effect also must be considered in evaluating the Experimental Group's scores on marital satisfaction. Although objective relationships were conscientiously maintained between the research team and the members of the Experimental Group, nevertheless there was more attention given to this group through the medium of follow-up telephone inquiries, whereas all communications with the subjects in the Control Group were done through the Lamaze teachers.

The major suggestions for further research include, of course, a larger sample size, with follow-up investigation at six months and one year postpartum. The research design could be considerably tightened by the addition of a second control group. In this group the subjects would be taught a different modality than Therapeutic Touch, one that elicits a deep relaxation response, in addition to having the Lamaze classes. Since a high rate of birth by caesarian section is reported nationwide (the statistics reported above of 24 percent caesarian births in New York City is not unusual in other large cities), a subset of this study could be run on couples whose children have been born in this manner. It also would be useful to look at various sociopsychological variables in replicated studies, such as changes in locus of control, strengthening of family cohesion, increase in social responsibility, and change in parenting role.

APPENDIX P

Therapeutic Touch During Childbirth Preparation: Explanation Offered to Persons Whose Permission is Requested

*T*he major purpose of this study is to collect information that will help nurses understand how touch affects married couples who have been trained in the Lamaze method of childbirth preparation for their first pregnancy. We are conducting this study through the use of questionnaires and personal interviews, which will be administered several times. The questionnaires will take about twenty minutes to fill out, and the interviews will take about the same time. In addition, we would like to teach the husbands a method for using their hands therapeutically on their wives during the pregnancy. To do this we will offer evening classes, which are open to the wives also.

During the course of the study we shall answer any questions you may wish to ask. Should you wish to, you may withdraw from the study at any time. The materials gathered for this study need not be identified with your name; for instance, you may use a code name or an imaginary name. The results of this study will be made available to you upon its completion at your request.

Thank you very much for your participation in this study.

Therapeutic Touch During Childbirth Preparation: Consent Form

*A*n explanation of the procedures to be used in the study has been offered to me. Also, I have been told an estimate of the time of my involvement in this study, and I've been given an overview of what I shall be asked to do. Questions that I have asked about the study have been answered to my satisfaction, and I know that I am free to withdraw from the study at any time. I understand that the data involved will remain confidential.

Signature: _____

Date: _____

Name (typed or printed):

_____

Study Number: _____

Investigator (type or print): _____

Signature: _____

Therapeutic Touch During Childbirth Preparation: Subjective Experience of Therapeutic Touch Scale (SETTS)

Patricia Winstead-Fry, Ph.D., R.N., and Dolores Krieger, Ph.D., R.N., New York University

The following sixty-eight items reflect experiences that Therapeutic Touch practitioners have had while performing Therapeutic Touch on healees. Not all of the experiences have been had by all practitioners. Depending on their length of experience and personal makeup, practitioners tend to experience the process differently, although there is an overall commonality in the larger context. This scale has been constructed to collect more specific information on the types of experiences and on the frequency with which they occur. Your individual response will be kept confidential. Please respond as honestly and as accurately as you can to each item.

INSTRUCTIONS

For each of the items, place a check mark in the column that corresponds to the frequency with which the experience occurs to you while you are engaged in the process of Therapeutic Touch. The columns are numbered; the significance of the numbers is as follows:

0—not at all 3—almost always

1—once in a while 4—all the time

2—frequently

At the top of page one you will find several spaces for filling in your age, sex, profession, and the number of months or years you have been practicing Therapeutic Touch. Please fill these in, but do not put your name on the form.

The items below are practice items.

Item Ranking

0	1	2	3	4	Healer's Experience of Therapeutic Touch
					I am aware of a part of my own being that is verbally or intuitively supplying me with a knowledge of the healee's illness.
					I feel the totality of beingness and openness to the healee and other people around me.

THERAPEUTIC TOUCH PRACTITIONER EXPERIENCE SURVEY

Age: _____ Sex: _____ Profession: _____

Months (Years) of Therapeutic Touch Practice _____

Questionnaire

Item Ranking					Experience of Therapeutic Touch by Healer
0	1	2	3	4	
					1. My heart and respiration rates feel slower.
					2. My breathing becomes slower and deeper.
					3. I feel sensations of heat and cold in my hands.
					4. I feel tingling sensations in my hands.
					5. I feel pressure in my hands.
					6. I feel electric shock sensations in my hands.
					7. I feel energy pulsations in my hands.
					8. I have the feeling that my hands are being spontaneously drawn to a particular area in the healee's field.
					9. I feel heat coming from my hands.
					10. I seem to be able to maintain uncomfortable postures much longer than usual.
					11. I seem to stand or kneel straighter than usual.
					12. My body movements become subtle, soft, and flowing.
					13. I become very sensitive to how I move my body and whether I am in an awkward or stressful position.

					Experience of Therapeutic Touch by Healer
Item Ranking					
0	1	2	3	4	
					14. My movements feel slow, steady, smooth, and alert.
					15. I feel energy moving through me and out of my hands.
					16. Energy flows more freely in my body.
					17. I get a sense of stillness and balance in my body, mind, and emotions.
					18. My body feels in harmony and seems to be an instrument through which energy flows.
					19. My body feels quiet, calm, and relaxed.
					20. I feel energy flowing rhythmically and evenly within my body.
					21. I feel physically balanced, lined up, or integrated.
					22. I feel as though my whole body is working in unison.
					23. I have a sense of physical and psychological attunement.
					24. All my senses are heightened and sharpened.
					25. I feel very close to the person I am healing.
					26. I feel impersonal love for the healee, regardless of whether I like the person before or not.
					27. I feel loving and accepting toward myself and the healee.
					28. I am more aware of my own emotions.

Item Ranking					Experience of Therapeutic Touch by Healer
0	1	2	3	4	
					29. My own emotions seem to be set aside during the healing process.
					30. I feel a sense of calmness, peace, and inner strength.
					31. I feel detached and purposeful.
					32. I feel an increase in sensitivity.
					33. I feel an increase in empathy.
					34. I feel an increase in compassion.
					35. Emotions of love and peace feel like waves of energy going through me to the healee.
					36. I am aware of the emotions of the healee as different qualities of energy.
					37. I feel joy.
					38. I trust that I have understanding at a level other than my conscious experience.
					39. I have a sense of the therapeutic touch process being a totally integrated, flowing interaction.
					40. I feel expansiveness.
					41. I see spontaneous mental images that let me know what is going on in the healee.
					42. I am most aware of the healee and less aware of activity going on in the surrounding environment.
					43. When I focus attention on my hands and my feelings, the external environment seems to recede.

Item Ranking					Experience of Therapeutic Touch by Healer
0	1	2	3	4	
					44. When I am focusing on the therapeutic touch process, my mind seems to split into one part that is primarily attending to the healing process and another part which simply remains in touch with events in the environment.
					45. My mental perception seems clearer during the therapeutic touch process.
					46. My thought processes seem to spring from intuitional insight rather than rationality.
					47. I have no thoughts during the therapeutic touch process.
					48. My thought processes seem to slow down.
					49. I have thoughts, but I don't attend to them unless they relate to the healee and the therapeutic touch process.
					50. My thoughts stop and intuitions, images, and impressions take over.
					51. I recognize imbalances in the healee's field.
					52. I am aware of consciously directing my attention inward in order to center myself as I start the therapeutic touch process.
					53. My sense of concentration increases.
					54. I am more aware of my inner being.
					55. I am not aware of time during the therapeutic touch process.

Item Ranking					Experience of Therapeutic Touch by Healer
0	1	2	3	4	
					56. I feel as if time stops.
					57. I feel as if time slows down.
					58. I feel as if time speeds up.
					59. While doing therapeutic touch, I feel that all personality patterns of the healee disappear and all I see is his or her inner beauty.
					60. I feel unified with the healee.
					61. My body feels like an expanding mass of energy.
					62. I feel as if my body is dissolving away and that I am becoming boundless.
					63. I experience my body as a continuous flow of energy rather than a set of distinct parts.
					64. My cognitive processes seem to step into the background and become secondary to a more intuitive process of knowledge.
					65. Parts of my body not actively involved in the therapeutic touch process feel heavy or nonexistent.
					66. I have a feeling of being united with the external environment.
					67. I have a sense of my own wholeness beyond my personality.
					68. I am aware of a part of my being that is verbally or intuitively supplying me with knowledge of how best to direct energies to the healee's field.

APPENDIX S

Therapeutic Touch During Childbirth Preparation: Protocol for Teaching Therapeutic Touch to Husbands

*T*he husbands were taught Therapeutic Touch in small groups while the married couples were attending Lamaze classes; that is, during the last trimester of pregnancy. The teaching was done by Krieger or a research assistant approved by her as an expert in Therapeutic Touch and its teaching. The teaching method was by lecture, audiovisual aid, demonstration, practicum, and discussion.

The audiovisual aid was a videotape specifically designed for this study by Krieger and Therese Connell-Meehan, Ph.D., R.N. The tape depicts a husband and his pregnant wife at home after having attended the workshop offered by this study's research team. The couple decides to practice the techniques they have just learned on how to combine Therapeutic Touch with childbirth preparation techniques. In the dialogue that follows they verbally reiterate the principles involved as they go through the various steps.

The sessions included a supervised practicum during which the husband demonstrated Therapeutic Touch techniques on his wife to the satisfaction of the person teaching the session. The formation of support groups among the husbands was encouraged and facilitated, and telephone numbers were exchanged between them.

Approximately one week after the teaching session, the research assistant telephoned each couple to find out how they had progressed with the techniques and if there were any questions. In the event that the husband was having difficulty with the techniques, the teacher met with the couple at the couple's convenience. The couples were free to call the research office for assistance with any aspect of Therapeutic Touch on any weekday. The Lamaze teachers assisted in this follow-up.

The husband was taught to use Therapeutic Touch on his wife during her pregnancy. He was asked to use these techniques at least two to three times a week and as needed, should there arise an occasion for which Therapeutic Touch was appropriate, such as nausea, headache, pain, sleeplessness, and so on. If there was, he was asked to let the obstetrician know of the intervention. Since there were no previous controlled studies on the treatment of pregnant women with Therapeutic Touch, it was decided to take a conservative stance. For this reason, it was requested that the husband not exceed ten minutes in the treatment of his wife with Therapeutic Touch and allow a minimum of two hours to elapse before repeating a treatment. There were no untoward effects reported in this sample, nor in subsequent small sample replications of this study. The protocol used for the Therapeutic Touch treatments was based on those developed by Krieger (see Chapter 1, note 12).

BASIC ASSUMPTIONS

Therapeutic Touch is a mode of energy transference for therapeutic purposes. This is based on a model of the human being as an open system of energy flow, as developed in the life sciences. The basic assumptions of the techniques derive from two sources: the life sciences and the world literature on healing.

One assumption is that physically humans have a bilateral symmetry. This can be most clearly seen in the skeleton, where there is a direct one-for-one reflection of bone for bone along the longitudinal axis of the body. A second assumption, held by healers in most cultures of the world, is that illness represents an imbalance of the energies in the human field. The techniques of Therapeutic Touch have been logically derived from these assumptions.

THERAPEUTIC TOUCH TECHNIQUE

The specific techniques used were the following.

The wife either sat in a chair or lay down on a bed or couch, whichever was the most comfortable position for her.

The husband took a few moments to center himself, either by a method he habitually used or in the following manner:

1. For a few moments he quieted himself by breathing slowly and fully in a normal manner.

2. He became aware of his state of consciousness during the natural pause between inhaling and exhaling, a sense of the stillness and quietude of his body.

3. He identified closely with that sense of quietude and gently, effortlessly tried to prolong that tranquil state of consciousness. He explored it as an experience in interiority, regardless of the phase of respiration.

4. He maintained that state of centeredness, breathing meanwhile in a quiet, normal manner, throughout the time that he was doing Therapeutic Touch to his wife. If for some reason he lost this sense of centeredness, he either stopped the treatment or he paused long enough to recenter himself.

The husband used the sensitivity of his hands to get a sense of the symmetrical relationship of his wife's energies, using the midline of her body as the reference for symmetry. Beginning at the crown of her head and keeping one hand on each side of the midline, about two to four inches from her body (a subjective decision), he moved his hands in a caudal (from head to feet) direction. Systematically he noted any difference he felt during the downward movement of his hands. He noted where he felt these differences in his wife's energy field.

He then redirected the energy bound up in those places where he had felt the differences by placing his hands either in direct body contact or just beyond the periphery of her body (another subjective decision) in an act of concentration. In a physically effortless manner he tried to change the quality of energy flow that characterized these areas by consciously directing to the region energy that had attributes of an opposite nature. For example, if the difference between one body area and its symmetrical opposite felt "hot" to his hands, he would visualize cold to himself and send a quality of energy akin to that feeling to the "hot" area in an attempt to "cool" it.* Based on an assumption that illness is an imbalance of energy, this was

---

*An analogy to the therapeutic use of opposites is in the way we use our emotions. For instance, we intentionally speak in a nonprovocative, hushed, and even manner if we wish to calm someone whose emotions are roiled in anger.

done in an attempt to restore the sense of balance with the energy tone of its symmetrical area.

The husband then reassessed the area in question in the manner noted above. If he no longer was aware of any differences in sensory cues, he could then logically assume that the wife's body energies were in balance, and he would terminate the procedure. If the sensory differences continued, he would again redirect the energies; however, under no circumstances did he continue treatment for more than ten minutes.

This technique rests on the guiding principle that Therapeutic Touch should not be continued without evidence that is helping the healee. The major indicators that Therapeutic Touch is useful are the onset of a relaxation response, a reduction or cessation of pain (should there have been complaints of pain), and the facilitation of the healing process.

In summary, it was operationally determined that the husband had learned Therapeutic Touch if he scored at least 30 points on the Subjective Experience of Therapeutic Touch Scale (SETTS). In addition, the husband's ability was checked individually in the practicum that followed the teaching session. One week after each practicum there were telephone interviews with each to discuss any difficulties in the use of Therapeutic Touch that may have arisen. If there were any problems, the investigator met with the husband and wife to clarify them. As noted in the report on this study, this situation arose only once.

NOTES

Introduction

‡ Dolores Krieger, *The Therapeutic Touch: How to Use Your Hands to Help or to Heal.* (Englewood Cliffs, New Jersey: Prentice-Hall, 1979).

Chapter 1

1. Gary E. Schwartz and Jackson Beatty, *Biofeedback: Theory and Research.* (New York: Academic Press, 1977).
2. Elmer Green and Alyce Green, *Beyond Biofeedback.* (New York: Dell Publishing, 1977), pp. 196–218.
3. Ibid, p. 218–25.
4. J.G. Miller, "Living Systems: Basic Concepts." *Behavioral Sciences* 10 (1965): 193.
5. Ludwig von Bertalanffy, *General Systems Theory.* (New York: Braziller, 1968).
6. Fritjof Capra, *The Tao of Physics.* (Berkeley: Shambhala, 1975).
7. Gary Zukav, *The Dancing Wu Li Masters.* (New York: William Morrow, 1979).
8. Kenneth R. Pelletier, *Mind as Healer, Mind as Slayer.* (New York: Delacorte, 1977).
9. Dolores Krieger, *The Foundations of Holistic Health Nursing Practices: The Renaissance Nurse.* (Philadelphia: J.B.Lippincott, 1981).
10. Herbert Benson, John F. Beary, and Mark P. Carol, "The Relaxation Response." *Psychiatry* 37 (1974): 37–46.

11. Marilyn Ferguson, *The Aquarian Conspiracy*. (Los Angeles: J.P.Tarcher, 1980).

12. Dolores Krieger, *The Therapeutic Touch: How to Use Your Hands to Help or to Heal*. (Englewood Cliffs, New Jersey: Prentice-Hall, 1979).

13. Ferguson, op.cit., p. 90.

14. Krieger (1979), op.cit., p. 76.

15. Krieger (1981), op.cit., p. 143.

16. Dolores Krieger, "The Relationship of Touch With the Intent to Help or to Heal, to Subjects' In-Vivo Hemoglobin Values: A Study in Personalized Interaction." *Proceedings of the Ninth American Nurses Association Nursing Research Conference*. (Kansas City: The Association, 1973).

17. Krieger, Dolores, "Therapeutic Touch: The Imprimatur of Nursing." *American Journal of Nursing* 75 (1975): 784–87.

18. Erik Peper and Sonia Ancoli, "The Two Endpoints of an EEG Continuum of Meditation." (Paper presented at the Biofeedback Society of America Research Conference, Orlando, Florida, March 1977).

19. Patricia Heidt, "Effects of Therapeutic Touch on Anxiety Levels of Hospitalized Patients." *Nursing Research* 30 (1981): 32–37.

20. Gretchen Randolph, "Therapeutic and Physical Touch: Physiological Response to Stressful Stimuli." *Nursing Research* 33 (1984): 33–36.

21. Janet Quinn, "The Effects of Therapeutic Touch Done Without Physical Contact on State Anxiety in Hospitalized Cardiovascular Patients." *Advances in Nursing Science* 6 (1984): 2.

22. Rosalie Fedoruk, "Transfer of the Relaxation Response: Therapeutic Touch as a Method of Reducing Stress in Premature Neonates." (Unpublished Ph.D. dissertation, University of Maryland, 1984).

23. Therese Connell-Meehan, "The Effect of Therapeutic Touch on the Experience of Acute Pain in Postoperative Patients." (Unpublished Ph.D. dissertation, New York University, 1985).

24. Harriet Lionberger, "An Interpretive Study of Nurses' Practice of Therapeutic Touch." (Unpublished Ns.Sc.D. dissertation, University of California/San Francisco, 1985).

25. Cecelia K. Ferguson, "Subjective Experience of Therapeutic Touch (SETTS): Psychometric Examination of an Instrument." (Unpublished Ph.D. dissertation, University of Texas/San Antonio, 1986).

26. Richard Katz, *Boiling Energy: Community Healing Among the Kalahari !Kung*. (Cambridge: Harvard University Press, 1982).

27. A.P. Elkin, *Aboriginal Men of High Degree*. 2d ed. (New York: St. Martin's Press, 1978).
28. Katz, op.cit., p. 225.
29. David Landy, *Culture, Disease and Healing: Studies in Medical Anthropology*. (New York: Macmillan, 1977), p. 415.
30. Octavio V. Romano, "Charismatic medicine, folk healing, and folk sainthood." *American Anthropologist* 67 (1965): 1151–73.
31. Brian Inglis, *Natural Medicine*. (Glasgow: William Collins, 1979).
32. T.H. Kuhn, *The Structure of Scientific Revolutions*. (Chicago: University of Chicago Press, 1962).
33. Abraham H. Maslow, *Toward a Psychology of Being*. (Princeton: Van Nostrand, 1962), pp. 91–95.

Chapter 2

34. Ira Progoff, *The Death and Rebirth of Psychology*. (New York: The Julian Press, 1956).
35. Krieger (1979), op.cit.
36. Abraham Maslow, *Motivation and Personality*. (New York: Harpers, 1954).
37. Abraham Maslow, *The Farther Reaches of Human Nature*. (New York: Viking, 1971).
38. Rollo May, *Love and Will*. (New York: Norton, 1969).
39. Silvano Arieti, *Creativity: The Magic Synthesis*. (New York: Basic Books, 1976).
40. Carl Jung, "On the Psychology of the Unconscious." In *The Collected Works of C. G. Jung*. vol. 7, *Two Essays on Analytical Psychology*. (Princeton: Princeton University Press, 1966), pp. 18–32.
41. Roberto Assagoli, *Psychosynthesis*. (New York: Viking, 1971).
42. *Histories of the Kings of Britain* trans. Sebastian Evans. (London: Dent, 1904).

Chapter 3

43. Jerome Frank, *Persuasion and Healing*. Rev. ed. (Baltimore: The Johns Hopkins University Press, 1973).
44. Dolores Krieger, Erik Peper, and Sonia Ancoli, "Physiological Indices of Therapeutic Touch." *American Journal of Nursing* 79 (1979): 660–62.

45. Mircea Eliade, *Patanjali and Yoga*. (New York: Schocken, 1975), p. 38.

46. Andras A. Anjyal, "A Theoretical Model for Personality Styles." In C. Moustakas, ed., *The Self: Explorations in Personal Growth*. (New York: Harper, 1956), pp. 44–45.

47. Claudio Naranjo, *The One Quest*. (New York: Viking, 1972), p. 138.

48. Lama A. Govinda, *Foundations of Tibetan Mysticism*. (London: Rider, 1969).

49. Ibid, p. 150.

50. *Conscious Multidimensionality*. (Wheaton: The Theosophical Publishing House, 1976), p. 136.

51. I. K. Taimini, *Gayatri: The Daily Religious Practice of the Hindus*. (Allahbad, India: The Ananda Publishing House, n.d.), p. 32.

52. Stanley Krippner and Alberto Villoldo, *Realms of Healing*. (Millbrae, California: Celestial Arts, 1976), p. 295.

53. Harry Edwards, *Psychic Healing*. (London: Spiritualist Press, 1952), p. 84.

54. Carl G. Jung, "Psychological commentary on Kundalini Yoga, Lecture IV." *Spring: An Annal of Archetypal Psychology and Jungian Thought*. (1976): 21, 27.

55. Arthur Avalon, *The Serpent Fire*. 7th ed. (Madras: Ganesh, 1964), pp. xi–xiv.

56. L. K. Yu, *The Secret of Chinese Meditation*. (London: Rider, 1964).

57. Gopi Krishna, *Kundalini: The Evolutionary Energy in Man*. (Berkeley: Shambhala, 1970).

58. Swami Ajaya, *Psychotherapy East and West: A Unifying Paradigm*. (Honesdale, Pennsylvania: The Himalayan Institute, 1983), p. 248.

59. Hiroshi Motoyama, *Theories of the Chakras*. (Wheaton: Theosophical Publishing House, 1981), p. 248.

60. Karlfried Durckheim, *Hara*. (London: Allen and Unwin, 1962), p. 24.

61. Motoyama, op.cit., p. 242.

62. Krippner and Villoldo, op.cit., pp. 25, 297–98.

63. Charles W. Leadbeater, *The Chakras*. (Wheaton: Theosophical Publishing House, 1974), p. 7.

64. Ken Wilber, *Up From Eden: A Transpersonal View of Human Evolution*. (Garden City: Doubleday, 1981), pp. 33–35.

65. Credo Vusa' Mazulu Mutwa, *My People*. (Tribridge, Kent: Peach Hall Works, 1969).

66. Jacob Needleman, *Consciousness and Tradition*. (New York: Crossroads, 1982).

Chapter 4

67. Josef Pieper, *Love and Inspiration: A Study of Plato's Phaedrus*. (London: Faber and Faber, 1965), p. 58.
68. Silvano Arieti, *Creativity: The Magic Synthesis*. (New York: Basic Books, 1976), pp. 405–410.
69. Stanley Marlan, "Depth Consciousness." In Valle and Eckartsberg, eds., *Metaphors of Consciousness*. (New York: Plenum, 1981), p. 238.
70. Michael Polanyi, *Tacit Dimension*.
71. Arieti, op. cit., pp. 54–61.
72. Krieger (1979), op. cit., pp. 50–51.
73. Marie Dellas and Eugene I. Gauer, "Identification of Creativity: The Individual." *Psychological Bulletin* 73 (1979): 55–73.
74. Carl Rogers, "Toward a Theory of Creativity." In H. H. Anderson, ed., *Creativity and its Cultivation*. (New York: Harper, 1954), pp. 69–82.

Chapter 5

75. C. Tart, "Physiological Correlates of Psi Cognition." *International Journal of Parapsychology* 5 (1965): 375–86.
76. D. Krieger, "Visualization by Professional Nurses During Meditation on Hospitalized Patients Who Are at a Distance." (Paper presented to Sigma Theta Tau, Alpha Zeta Chapter, University of Texas/Houston, April 10, 1981).
77. R. Targ and H. E. Puthoff, "Information Transfer Under Conditions of Sensory Shielding." *Nature* 252 (1974): 602–607.
78. H. E. Puthoff and R. Targ, "A Perceptual Channel for Information Transfers over Kilometer Distances: Historical Perspectives and Recent Research." *Proceedings of the Institute of Electrical and Electronic Engineers* 64 (1976): 329–54.
79. "Science and the Citizen." *Scientific American* (1979): 240–84.
80. A. L. Edwards, *Statistical Methods for the Behavioral Sciences*. (New York: Holt, Rinehart and Winston, 1963), pp. 472–76.
81. Ibid, p. 69.
82. J. Achterberg and G. F. Lawton, *Imagery of Cancer*. (Champaign, Illinois: Institute for Personality and Ability Testing, 1978).
83. D. Boyd, *Rolling Thunder*. (New York: Delta, 1974).

Chapter 6

84. Cherie Burns, "Healing with the Hands: The Medical Mystery of Therapeutic Touch." *Glamour*, June 1983, p. 60.

Chapter 7

85. Hans Selye, *Stress Without Distress*. (Philadelphia: J.B. Lippincott, 1974).
86. M. Murphy, "The Body." In *Millennium*. (Boston: Houghton-Mifflin, 1981), p. 82.
87. D. Wheatley, "Evaluation of Psychotropic Drugs in General Practice." *Proceedings of the Royal Society of Medicine* 65 (1972): 317.
88. W. Evans and C. Hoyle, "The Comparative Value of Drugs Used in the Continuous Treatment of Angina Pectoris." *Quarterly Journal of Medicine* (July 1973), pp. 311–38.
89. B. Inglis, *The Diseases of Civilization*. (London: Hodder and Stoughton, 1981), pp. 284–88.

Appendix F

90. J. Piaget, *The Origin of Intelligence in Children*. (New York: International Press, 1952).
91. A. Luria, *The Mind of a Mnemonist*. (New York: Basic Books, 1968).
92. J. Khatina, "Vividness in Imagery and Creative Self Perception." *The Gifted Child Quarterly* 19 (1975): 33–37.
93. R. Wagman and C. Stewart, "Vivid Imagery and Hypnotic Susceptibility." *Perceptual and Motor Skills* 38 (1974): 815–22.
94. J. Schultz and W. Luthe. *Autogenic Training: A Psychophysiologic Approach to Psychotherapy*. (New York: Grune and Stratton, 1959).
95. E. E. Green, A. M. Green, and E. D. Walters, "Voluntary Controls of Internal States: Psychological and Physiological." *Journal of Transpersonal Psychology* 2 (1970): 1–26.
96. O.C. Simonton, S. Matthew-Simonton, and J. Creighton, *Getting Well Again*. (New York: St. Martin's Press, 1978).
97. V. Neisser, "The Process of Vision." In *Perception: Mechanisms and Models*. (San Francisco: W. H. Freeman, 1972).
98. G. Trowbridge, *Swedenborg: Life and Teachings*. (London: Swedenborg Society, 1945).
99. J. B. Rhine, *New Frontiers of Mind*. (New York: Farrar and Rinehart, 1937).
100. J. Pratt, J. B. Rhine, and L. Rhine, *Extra-Sensory Perception After Sixty Years*. (New York: Henry Holt, 1940).

101. S. G. Soal and F. Bateman, *Modern Experiments in Telepathy*. (London: Faber and Faber, 1953).

102. E. D. Dean, "Plethysmograph Recordings in ESP Response." *International Journal of Neuropsychiatry* 2 (1966): 121–23.

103. G. E. Schwartz, Towards a Theory of Voluntary Control Response Patterns in the Cardiovascular System." In P. A. Obrist, A. H. Black, and L. V. Dicara, eds., *Cardiovascular Psychophysiology*. (Chicago: Aldine Press, 1974).

104. D. H. Doyd, "Objective Events in the Brain Correlating with Psychic Phenomena." *New Horizons* 2 (Summer 1973): 2.

105. R. E. Ornstein, *The Mind Field*. (New York: Grossman, 1976), p. 68.

Appendix J

106. Fernand Lamaze, *Painless Childbirth: The Psychoprophylactic Method*. L. R. Celestin, trans. (Chicago: Contemporary Books, 1970).

107. E. Bing, *Six Practical Lessons for an Easier Childbirth: The Lamaze Method*. (New York: Bantam Books, 1978).

Appendix K

108. P. Winstead-Fry and D. Krieger, *Subjective Experience of Therapeutic Touch: An Evaluation Tool for Three Levels of Healing*. (In press.)

109. D. Krieger, "Therapeutic Touch During Childbirth Preparation by the Lamaze Method and Its Relation to Marital Satisfaction and State Anxiety of the Married Couple." (*Proceedings Research Day*, Sigma Theta Tau, Upsilon Chapter, New York University, November 7, 1984).

110. C. Hoskins and P. R. Merrifield, *Interpersonal Conflict Scale*. (Saluda, North Carolina: Family Life Publications, 1980).

111. C. D. Spielberger, R. L. Gorsuch, and R. E. Lushene, *STAI Manual for the State-Trait Inventory*. (Palo Alto: Consulting Psychologists Press, 1970).

Appendix N

112. D. Moore, "Prepared Childbirth and Marital Satisfaction." *Nursing Research* 32 (1983): 2:73–79.

Appendix O

113. Heidt, op. cit.

114. Quinn, op. cit.

INDEX

A

Ajaya, Swami, 45, 47, 49, 52
Anandamayakosha, 59
Archetypes, 17, 45
  archetypal themes and chakras
    anja chakra, 47, 50
    anahata chakra, 49
    Child, The, 49
    Hedonist, The, 48
    Hero, The, 49
    Sage, The, 50
    Savior, The, 49
    Victim, The, 47
Asanas, 47
Assessment
  description of process, 105–6
  intuition, testing, 25
  looking into distance and, 106
  nonlogical basis for, 68–69
  and reassessment, 106
Australian aboriginal healers, 9
Autogenic training, 35–36, 136
Autosuggestion, 35, 118, 119, 136
  See also Placebo response.

B

Biofeedback, 2, 136
  research findings, 141
Bodhisattva, 18
Breathing exercises, chakras,
    awakening, 47
Buddhism, and yoga, 40

C

Chakras 9, 43
  ajna chakra, 47, 50
  anahata chakra, 49
  archetypal themes
    Child, The, 49
    Hedonist, The, 48
    Hero, The, 49
    Sage, The, 50
    Savior, The, 49
    Victim, The, 47
  awakening of, 47
    Indian method, 47
  healing, use in, 52–53
  higher chakras, 50
    location of, 46–47
  Jungian model, 44, 45
  level of functioning, 9
  lower chakras, location of, 47
  manipura chakra, 48, 49
  muladhara chakra, 47
  and nonhumans, communication
    with, 55–58
  and paranormal states, 78
  psychotherapeutic view, 45–46
  sahasrara chakra, 50
  svadhisthana chakra, 47–48, 49
  and Therapeutic Touch, study
    of, 53
  vishuddha chakra, 49
Ch'i, 8, 52
Child, The, archetypal theme, cha-
    kras, 49
Childbirth preparation Therapeutic
    Touch study, 109–10, 157–87

Childbirth preparation Therapeutic
(Cont.)
consent form, 176
definition of terms, 159–60
delimitations of study, 161
hypothesis, 161–62
literature review, 164–66
methodology, 167–70
research question, 162
results/discussion, 170–74
significance of study, 163
Subjective Experience Therapeutic
Touch Scale, 177–83
teaching techniques for husbands,
184–87
Complementarity, Heisenberg's
principle of, 1
Consciousness, Hindu view of, 59–60
Creativity and healing
creative listening, 67
encouragement of, 73
flash of inspiration, 68
healer as creative person, 69–73
Credo Uusa' Mazulu Mutwa, 54–55
interview with, 54–55
Curandero, 10

D

Darsana, 43
Depth psychology, 66
Development
of touch, 103–4
of visualization, 136
Dhen Wantari, 11
Dragon Project, 30–31, 32
findings of, 31

E

Edwards, Harry, 43
Ego structure, changes in, 66–67
Emotions
origins of, 59
and psychodynamic field, 58–60,
61–62
psychosomatic effects, 62
Endocepts, 67
Energy, 127
energy flow, 36–37, 42–43
forms of, 127

visualization of forms, 127–28
repatterning of, 37–38, 116

G

Galen, 11
Greatrakes, Valentine, 11–12
Guided imagery, 36

H

Hadrian, 11
Hand chakras, 105
Hara, 48
Healers
as "channel" for healing, 39
characteristics of, 125
clues to illness for, 75, 76
and creative person, similarity to,
69–73
effect of healing on, 16
healing experience, 38–39
historical view, 10–12
inner changes in early stages,
22–23
intentionality and, 23
interiority of, 9–10, 26
intuition of, 24–26
motivation to heal, 23–24
novice healer, 18–21
case examples, 19–22
feelings of, 18–19
personality patterns of, 39
self-awareness tool for, 126
senses, use of, 75–76
temperament of, 3
wounded healer, 17–18
views of, 18
Healing
at a distance, 79–81
experiment in, 79–81
visualization experiment, 82–102
creativity, 65–73
creative listening, 67
encouragement of, 73
flash of inspiration, 68
healer as creative person, 69–73
similarities in, 66
descriptions of healing process,
50–52
dynamics of, 6–9

effect of study on researchers, 1
ego structure in, 66–67
energy
   energy flow in, 36–37, 42–43
   repatterning of, 37–38, 116
healer/healee responses, 67
   emotional response, 71
historical view, 8, 9–10
as a lifestyle, 123
ordering principles of, 122–23
perceptions, repatterning of, 38–39
research studies, 12–16
   blood analysis study, 13–14
self-healing, 34–35
   innate bodily healing and, 35
   tissues capable of, 36
timing and, 13, 14
   importance of, 14, 15
as yoga, 38, 39–50
   energy systems in, 42–43
   healer's experience and, 42–43
   healer's worldview, 44
   healing as lifestyle perspective, 43
   pranic flow, in, 43–44
   similarities in, 43–44
Health, and needs theory, 22
Hedonist, The, archetypal theme, chakras, 48
Hero, The, archetypal theme, chakras, 49
Hippocrates, 11
Holistic health, focus of, 3–4

I

Ida, 47
Illness
   definition of, 35
   stress, effects of, 117
Interiority, of healers, 9–10, 26
Intuition
   activation of, 24
   and assessment method of therapeutic touch, 25
   development of, 32
   of healer, 24–26
   Jungian model, 24
Izinyanga, 9

J

Japanese, hara, 48
Jesus Christ, 11
Jungian models
   archetypes, 17
   chakra system, 44, 45
   intuition, 24

K

Ka, 8
Kosha, 59
Kundalini, 7, 47
   basis of, 44
Kunz, Dora, 7

L

Laying-on of hands, 7

M

Mana, 8
Manambal, 9
Mandalas, as focusing aids, 122–23
Manipura chakra, 48, 49
MEDLINE, 8
Metaneeds, 22
Mudras, 47
Muladhara chakra, 47

N

Nabhisthana chakra, 49
Nadis, 8, 44
Needs theory
   Metaneeds, 22
   Self-actualization, 16
New consciousness, stages in
   entry point, 4
   exploration, 4–5
   integration, 5
New Testament, healing, references to, 11
Nonhumans, psychic communication with, 55–58
Novice healer, 18–21
   case examples, 19–22
   feelings of, 18–19
NUM, 10

Nurses
  attrition rate, 95
  visualization experiment, implications for, 95–96

P

Patanjali, 40
Perceptions, repatterning of, 38–39
Pingala, 47
Placebo response, 36
  double-blind studies, 119
  effects of, 118
  power of, 118
  as self-healing, 121
Prana, 7, 8, 9
  pranic flow, 43–44
  and spleenic chakra, 48–49
Pranamayakosha, 59
Pranayamas, 47
Pregnancy, fathers and Therapeutic Touch, 109–10
  See also Childbirth preparation, Therapeutic Touch Study.
Psi, 82
Psychic gates, chakras, awakening, 47, 49
Psychodynamic field
  conscious use of, 60–63
  and emotions, 61–62
  exercises
    exploration of another's field, 131–32
    exploration of one's field, 129–30
    human field holomovement, 134–35
  main characteristic of, 59
  sensitivity of, 61
  unrestrained, instances of, 60
Psychokinesis, *svadhisthana* chakra, 48
Psychosomatic illness, 117
  and emotions, 62
Purnananda, 44

R

Reality
  basis for, 75
  East/West view, 40
Rollright stone circle site, 27

Dragon Project, 30–31, 32
  findings of, 31
  impressions of, 27–29
  possible purpose of, 31–32

S

Sage, The, archetypal theme, chakras, 50
Sahasrara chakra, 50
St. Bernard, 11
St. Patrick, 11
Savior, The, archetypal theme, chakras, 49
Self-actualization, 16
Self-awareness tool, for healers, 126
Self-healing, 5, 34–35
  empowering the patient, 121–22
  innate bodily healing and, 35
  placebo response as, 121
  tissues capable of, 36
Senses of healer
  latent senses, fostering, 77–78
  use of, 75–76
Siddhis, 82
Spleenic chakra, 48–49
  and *prana*, 48–49
Stonehenge, as healing site, 32
Stress
  effects of, 117
  and rise of therapeutic modes, 3
Sushumna, 47
Svadhisthana chakra, 47–48, 49
  psychokinesis, 48
Swedenborg, Emmanuel, 137
Systems theory, 3

T

Tension, definition of, 35
Therapeutic Touch
  assessment method, 25
  basis of, 7, 8
  versus laying-on of hands, 7, 8
  See also individual topics.
Third eye, 47
Thrita, 11
Timing
  and healing, 13, 14, 15
  importance of, 14, 15
Touch

development of, 103–4
non-contact touch experiment,
   107–12
   implications of, 110–12
   pilot study, 108–10
in Therapeutic Touch, 104–7
   description of process, 105
Transference, 71

V

Vespasian, 11
Victim, The, archetypal theme,
   chakras, 47
Vijnanamayakosha, 59
Visualization
   cross-cultural view, 82
   development of, 136
   as intrapsychic event, 137
      example of, 137
   nurses/patients, case examples, 97–
      101
   paradox related to, 83, 136
   studies of
      card guessing studies, 137
      eidetic imagery, 136
      plethysmograph, use in, 138
      principal findings, 140
      psi cognition studies, 138–39
      remote viewing studies, 139
      statistical analysis, 142–46
Visualization experiment, 82–102
   data analysis, 91
   data-collection instruments, 87–88
   hypothesis in, 85–86
   implications for professional
      nursing, 95–96

objectives of, 83–84
pilot study, 82
procedures used, 88–91
random assignment, 87
reliability/validity, 88
results of study, 91–95
sample characteristics, 86
terms used, definitions, 84–85
Vivid visualization, *See also* Visualization; Visualization
   experiment.

W

Wa Na, 10
Wounded healer, 17–18
   views of, 18

Y

Ylun, 8
Yoga
   chakras, 41, 44–50
   as healing
      energy systems in, 42–43
      healer's experience and, 42–43
      healer's worldview, 44
      healing as lifestyle perspective, 43
      pranic flow in, 43–44
      similarities in, 43–44
   and healer's experience, 42–43
   origin of term, 39
   physical body in, 41
   purpose of, 40, 42
   relationship to Buddhism, 40
   secret of, 40
   teachings, basis of, 40–41